THE MAGIC OF
CHIA

REVIVAL OF AN ANCIENT WONDER FOOD

JAMES F. SCHEER

Frog, Ltd.
Berkeley, California

The Magic of Chia

Published by Frog, Ltd.
Frog, Ltd. books are distributed by
North Atlantic Books
P.O. Box 12327
Berkeley, CA 94712

Cover and book design © Ayelet Maida, A/M Studios
Printed in the United States of America

Library of Congress Cataloging-in-Publication Data

Scheer, James F.
   The magic of Chia: revival of an ancient wonder food/by James Scheer.
      p. cm.
   ISBN 1-58394-040-5 (trade paper: alk. paper)
   1. Chia   I. Title

TX558.C38 S34 2000
641.3'56—dc21
      00-063633

1   2   3   4   5   6   7   8   9   /   05   04   03   02   01

Dedication

For my wife Joan Davidson-Scheer:
All of my love is gift-wrapped for you.

—Jim

Contents

Preface

ONE OF THE BEST-KEPT SECRETS IN NUTRITION IS THE SEED OF a desert plant called chia, among the most nourishing, energy-giving, endurance-sustaining food products ever discovered. There are good reasons why it is such a secret, as will be explained later.

Toward the end of the twelfth century, long before the New World got in the way of an India-bound explorer named Christopher Columbus, chia seed was already an important food there.

Cherished by a succession of Aztec emperors, chia was second only to corn and beans in importance as a food crop, with amaranth rated after chia. It was eaten as a seed, ground into flour, used as a medicine and pressed into oil.[1]

Royal planters of Aztec emperors grew precious chia seeds in "floating gardens" surrounding their capital city of Tenochitlan. The Aztecs created the novel idea of growing flowers, decorative plants, chia, and other foods on numerous soil-covered rafts floating on a shallow lake. Eventually, these rafts became small islands rooted to the lake bottom.[2]

Breaking the Royal Monopoly

Initially products from the floating gardens and the rich soil in the emperor's extensive and well-guarded land holdings were his exclusive property.

Legends tell us that all Aztec classes—nobility, healers, the military and merchants, and crop growers, reluctant to accept the royal monopoly on chia, smuggled chia plants out of the royal domain. Over the centuries they were cultivated throughout the Aztec empire.

Soon chia seed became a staple food in the marketplace. The emperor's subjects paid their annual tribute to him, a form of taxes, with chia seed. In time, chia seed became legal tender.

As archaeologists have discovered, chia seed was buried in the graves of Aztec and Mayan emperors, just as favorite foods were placed in the tombs of Egyptian pharaohs. Chia seeds were so important to the Aztecs that they served as an offering to their deity Chicome Coatl.

In the early 1500s Hernando Cortez, leading the Spanish conquerors, subjugated the proud Aztecs, under Emperor Montezuma, with a combination of diplomacy, deceit, cunning and superior weapons.

Impressed with the energy, endurance, and vitality derived from eating chia seeds, Cortez sent chia plants back to Spain, where they were neither appreciated nor cultivated.

Chia Spoken Here!

Chia seed actually became a part of the Aztec's language, as revealed in the twelve-volume *Florentine Codex,* written by Father Bernardino de Sahagun between 1558 and 1569. After mentioning that some types of chia seed were golden brown and speckled, Fr. Sahagun wrote that a common butterfly was characterized by the Aztecan term *chian papoloti.* The butterfly is painted "as if sprinkled with chia, flecked everywhere on its body, and its wings are painted, painted with the chia design."[3]

According to the *Florentine Codex*, the Aztecs made dough called *tzaoll* in the likeness of the goddess Chicome Coatl in the courtyard of her pyramid. To her they offered all varieties of maize, all varieties of beans, and all varieties of chia. This was because she was "the maker and giver of all those things which are necessaries of life, that people may live."

Father Knows Best

Fr. Sahagun's account of chia's use as a food is colorful and quaint:

"Everyone knows how atole is made." (Not I, father!) Then he writes that parched maize kernels are mixed with chia seed, a savory food. Ground raw, a little—half the length of the little finger—is mixed with opossum tail and water. If this is drunk by the woman about to give birth, she will promptly deliver her child.

Fr. Sahagun writes that the gelatinous chia seed—without opossum tail—is drunk during fasting and clears the chest. Also, it is like atole when mixed with grains of maize or with toasted tortillas.

When the oil is pressed or squeezed out of chia seed, painters apply it and beautify their work. It can be used like a varnish to make picture frames or furniture glossy, he writes.[4]

How It Looks, Where It Grows

Perhaps the most widespread and best known variety of chia is *Salvia hispanica,* an annual plant with a four-sided, almost square stem, bearing oval leaves. Blue flowers sprout from long spikes at the end of the branches. Four seeds rest in the base of the plant's calyx, a green outer whorl. Another common and prolific chia grows in areas with deep, sandy clay soils: the *Columbariae*.

Thanks to the Aztecs' love of chia, other neighboring Indian cultures throughout Mexico and in what is now the southwestern United States began harvesting and eating chia, which grows wild and abundantly in sandy and desert soil under 4,000 feet altitude.

Enough to Go Around

Thanks also to the Aztecs, Mayas, Tehuantapecs and Native Americans, we owe the information that chia seed is one of nature's few near-complete foods.

Use of chia seed by Native Americans helped point the way for two southern Californians—Bob Andersen, of Valley Center, and Hal Neiman, of Santa Monica—to spend nearly twenty years cultivating the most health-beneficial forms of chia seed and growing them in vast amounts so that, for the first time, there is enough chia seed to meet the mounting worldwide demand.

This book is a salute to Andersen and Neiman for their vision, faith, diligence, patience, persistence, and heavy investment of money in cultivating chia from the wild state to domesticity!

Acknowledgments

THOMAS JEFFERSON HAD IN MIND A PERSON SUCH AS BOB Andersen when he wrote, "No service can be rendered to a country that is more valuable than to introduce a new plant to the culture."

Actually, Bob and partner Hal Neiman did more than introduce a new plant. They domesticated a wild plant whose seeds were a staple food of the pre-Columbian Aztecs, Mayas, Tehuantepecs, and Indians of the desert southwest of what is now the United States. Chia seed imparted high energy, endurance, and good health to these people. In modern times chia plants grow mainly in the wild state.

Bob Andersen risked precious time, energy, and a considerable investment to domesticate the wild chia—a plant with the heavy advantage of being able to thrive with minimal water. Bob's initial goal was to supply enough chia seed for the United States and, in time, the rest of the world. He can now supply the United States. Over twenty years of chia domestication, Bob learned many things—often the hard way—about growing the chia plant, its value as a food, and its colorful history. I'm eternally grateful for the information he gathered for two decades and generously shared with me for the writing of this book and also for his guidance in this endeavor.

Bob and Hal Neiman also met 102-year-old Harrison Doyle, a chia growing expert and historian who had lived among Native Americans and witnessed dramatic results gained from eating chia seed daily. They interviewed him for information about his long relationship with American Indians and their and his use of chia seed.

Clyde Hogan, of Paso Robles, California, who spent much time with Doyle and interviewed him in depth, relayed a great deal more information to me over a half day's time.

A debt of gratitude to nutrition pioneer Paul Bragg cannot be repaid to him on this plane. Decades ago, when I heard his lecture on the powerful influence of chia seed on his body, mind, and spirit, I never thought I would ever write about this food, because it was rarely available in nutrition centers. However, his daughter Patricia, who is carrying on the Bragg tradition and nutrition business, will hear thanks from me.

My friend Francis M. Pottenger, Jr., M.D., one of the first medical doctors to prescribe food and supplements rather than drugs, first excited my interest in chia seed. It warms me to think that his memory lives on through the Price-Pottenger Foundation, in greater San Diego, directed by Patricia Connolly.

The same goes for Weston Price, D.D.S., the Cleveland dentist who in the 1930s studied cultures in primitive pockets of the world and proved with words and photos that processed foods are destroying the teeth and health of natives. Almost a generation ago, I met Dr. Price through his classic book, *Nutrition and Physical Degeneration.* He taught me the high value of natural foods.

In his offices on Hollywood's Sunset Strip, W. Coda Martin, M.D., another great man of medicine far ahead of the times, pointed me toward chia seed and other super health foods.

Sage counsel in how to write this book came from Hal Neiman during much of the chia seed adventure.

And speaking of counsel, James Brown, president of International Flora Technologies, and chia researcher Robert Kleiman, of the same organization, generously offered research information and priceless advice.

Linda Barrett and Bill Anderson, of Paso Robles, California, created and tested the chia recipes in this book and permitted me to use them. They deserve a resounding thank you, as well as a sharp salute for their idealism in working with the Paso Robles School District to upgrade school lunches to enhance student learning and memory and to offer a pilot program for school districts throughout the nation to follow.

My wife, Joan Davidson-Scheer, combed the Internet for chia information used in various chapters. I can't thank her enough for her encouragement and her sound advice and guidance in the writing of *The Magic of Chia*.

A person who doesn't even know she helped me in creating this book is the late Barbara Cartland, England's first lady of nutrition and the author of *The Magic of Honey*, a multimillion best-seller, as well as more romance novels than anyone else in the world. Some years ago, during tea at her manor in Hatfield, north of London, she suggested that I write a book about a key health food and use the word "magic" in the title. My deepest gratitude, Barbara. I would also like to thank Jennifer Privateer for her thoughtful editing and good humor in getting this book produced.

Dozens of research sources cited in references supplied invaluable help to me in the writing.

Last and far from least, thanks to my dear friend and coauthor of many books, booklets, articles, and columns, Stephen Langer, M.D., of Berkeley, California, who is younger than I but, in wise counsel, always "my big brother."

These thanks could go on from here to eternity, but there's a world of chia seed information to be shared in the pages that follow. So, on with the book! —James F. Scheer

CHAPTER 1

The Secret Is Out

ANCIENT HISTORY RAN SMACK INTO MODERN HISTORY A FEW years ago when Ciraldo Chacarito, a fifty-two-year-old Tarahumara Indian from the Copper Canyon region of Mexico, was among the top finishers in a 200-mile race.

This was phenomenal, because Ciraldo competed against the world's best young endurance runners with daily access to the latest training facilities, leading trainers, and scientifically designed running equipment.

Ciraldo hadn't conditioned himself. It was just "come as you are" to him. His competitors wore ultramodern running footwear designed for speed, rather than native, hand-made sandals like Ciraldo's.

Could the secret to Ciraldo's success have been something known for more than eight hundred years by his people: chia seeds eaten before and during the race? Teams of Tarahumara Indians are now training on chia seed, including Ciraldo, who won this race in 1998.

How It Does What It Does

Ciraldo hasn't the vaguest idea why chia works, only that it works—and always has for his people. Today biochemists know some of the whys. Chia seeds absorb seven times their weight in water and form a gel that causes a slow release of carbohydrates and an equally slow conversion of carbohydrates into sugar for energy.

Rich in the essential fatty acids omega-3 and omega-6, chia seeds supply many of the raw materials for forming the walls of our trillions of cells, making them soft and pliable, offering easy entry for oxygen and nutrients to supply energy and body heat and easy exit for carbon dioxide and wastes.

Athletes in competitive events where super energy and endurance are needed include omega-3 and omega-6 essential fatty acids in their supplements.

Worth Talking About

Until the news media revealed the potential of chia seed, the world hadn't heard much about it. It was not that the world was hard of hearing, it was just that few people were talking about chia seed and why it imparts special strength and endurance to those who eat it.

After all, there wasn't enough chia seed around to talk about—let alone to market. Growing wild in remote desert and low mountainous areas, chia was not financially feasible to harvest.

After he had eaten chia seed and was amazed at his physical response to it, Bob Andersen, a health food distributor in Valley Center, California, told himself, "Somebody ought to domesticate chia seed, develop a cost-effective way to harvest it, and assure a steady market supply for the world."

Nobody did it, so Bob Andersen became that somebody, along with his friend Hal Neiman. (I'll talk more about Bob and his uphill battle to make chia market-available in a later chapter. Another person, Ralph Rischman, also recently joined the chia team.)

From Skeptic to Believer

There were skeptics who wondered how such little seeds could make such a big difference in energy and endurance.

One of them was Milos Sarcev (pronounced MEElosh SHARchev). Milos was Iron Man champion of then Yugoslavia and a winner of first, second, and third place awards for body-building competitions like Mr. Universe and others that catapulted Arnold Schwarzenegger to filmdom fame.

In a telephone interview, Milos, who owns and operates the Powerhouse Gym, a body-building establishment in Fullerton (Orange County), California, told me, "I had never heard of chia seed a year ago. Then Bob Andersen gave me a manuscript copy of this book, and I was impressed. He also gave me samples of chia seed. These are a real blessing.

A Vote of Confidence

"I train daily for at least two hours, and these seeds turn out to be a perfect food for body-builders—any athletes, for that matter—and people in general.

"Chia seed is truly a renaissance food. I take it every day, and my energy and endurance levels are sky-high. Chia seed contains protein, the essential amino acids, fiber, calcium, and other major minerals, as well as essential fatty acids (EFAs)—that is, acids the body can't produce. They contain more EFAs and a more favorable ratio of omega-3 to omega-6 oil than flax seed oils.

"For more than a year, I have been dissolving three or four tablespoons of the chia seed in water, then spreading that amount on my breakfast oatmeal or adding it to my protein drink.

"Chia seed is such a nutritional asset that I recommend it to those who work out in my gym. I'm getting great feedback from those who try it. They're experiencing a marked physical boost and the extra endurance that I am."

Beyond Energy and Endurance

However, benefits from chia seed are not limited to energy and endurance, important as those are. There are numerous other health benefits.

Not long ago, *New York Times* nutrition columnist Jane E. Brody wrote a revealing article about the Arizona Native Americans and their effort to preserve their health by reclaiming ancient foods—chia seeds among them.[1]

The subhead of the article reads, "Desert's Bounty Beats Overweight and Diabetes." Here are the most significant points of this article:

These foods may prove valuable to non-Indians susceptible to overweight and diabetes and, perhaps, to those prone to high blood pressure and heart disease.

Benefits found in more familiar foods like oat bran and okra proceed from two characteristics of the native foods chia, cholla, and mesquite. Their high content of soluble fibers that form edible gels, gums, and mucilages and a type of starch called amylose are digested very slowly.

"The combined effect is to prevent wide swings in blood sugar, slow down the digestive process, and delay the return of hunger," writes Brody. "Peaks in blood sugar increase the body's need for insulin, and drops in blood sugar can bring on feelings of hunger.

"In the form of diabetes that strikes these Indians, their overweight bodies become insensitive to insulin, and slow digestion diminishes the need for insulin," she concludes.

There's much more to the story of chia seeds, their health benefits, and history. I was fortunate to be a small part of the revival of this ancient wonder food.

CHAPTER 2

Chia: A Seed of Greatness

I HAD HEARD MANY FASCINATING FACTS ABOUT CHIA SEED while editor of *Let's Live* magazine some years ago. During this period I received an unsolicited sales pitch for it from an assistant manager of a health food store in Arcadia (southern California), where I was buying vitamins.

This electrically charged, enthusiastic, semibalding, seemingly middle-aged man asked me if I had ever eaten chia seeds.

"Just samples," I replied.

"It's the most remarkable food I've ever encountered," he said. "For about twenty years, I have been mixing it with whole-grain cereals, the batter for waffles and pancakes, scrambled eggs—even hamburgers—and I feel great. Guess how old I am?" Then, scowling, he warned, "Don't try to flatter me!"

I studied him, noting his smooth, almost glowing pink skin, just a hint of grey in his sideburns, his slender figure and crackling energy.

"About fifty-one."

He laughed an ear-splitting laugh.

"I'm seventy-two and feel like a kid. I attribute it mainly to chia, although I also eat brewer's yeast, wheat germ, desiccated liver, and yogurt with natural, nutrient-rich foods."

Then, tapping a tanned forefinger on a tall apothecary glass full of small, dark brown seeds, he leaned across the counter and insisted:

"You ought to write an article about chia for *Let's Live.*"

"It would be unfair to excite reader interest when there's rarely enough chia seed to satisfy demand," I responded.

"That's true," he replied. "Harvesting wild chia in the desert is a long and costly process, and nobody seems to do it regularly."

That was more than twenty years ago, and I've thought a lot about chia since then. My interest in it soared to a new high not long ago, when I attended the Natural Products Expo in Anaheim, California, and by sheer chance met a friendly, positive-spirited gentleman named Bob Andersen in one of the many display booths. He represented the American Kamut Association, which promotes use of the exotic grain kamut. I introduced myself.

"Your name's familiar," he told me. "Haven't you done a lot of writing on nutrition?"

"A couple million words in books and magazine articles. Editing of health magazines, as well."

A Pertinent Contradiction

After talking about how popular kamut had become, Andersen said, "It's too bad so little has been written about chia seed."

"That's because so little chia is available."

"Oh, no!" Andersen corrected me. "Not anymore. Hal Neiman and I have been domesticating the most nutritious kinds of chia seed for almost two decades. We're growing it in abundance in Central and South America."

Surprised, I replied,

"Great. I've wanted to write about chia seed for ages."

"Be my guest," said Andersen. "I'll let you borrow research material I've taken decades to gather."

That's how I began to research chia seed in agricultural and ethnobiological reports, reference books, and personal interviews and how this book came to be written.

A lot of information for it was supplied through Bob Andersen and Hal Neiman's conversations with Harrison Doyle, of Vista, California, who was 102 years old at the start of this book's writing. No longer alive, Doyle studied and experimented with growing and eating of various varieties of chia seed in many recipes for most of his life. He attributed his amazing longevity to chia seed.[1]

Many millions of people know about chia seed without realizing that it is a potent food. They are familiar with a novelty product, the ceramic Chia Pet.

The Chia Pet is soaked in a basin of water overnight. Chia seeds are also soaked in water, but only until they become slightly gelatinous. They are then applied to the sides of the animal. Soon green "fur" sprouts from the seeds. The Chia Pet is an excellent means of introducing chia seed to the world and demonstrates that it can be sprouted for eating by individuals who know the super nutritional value of sprouts.

Beyond the Chia Pet

Now that the Chia Pet has brought joy to children for more than a decade, Bob Andersen wants the world to know that the seed can also bring abundant health to people of all ages.

Many sensational stories about chia seed are repeated by Native American tribes in the great Southwest, as recounted by Harrison Doyle. Most of them relate to the strength and endurance imparted by chia. It was nothing for tribesmen to run for an entire day on a handful of chia seeds and a gourd filled with water.

Legend and Folklore

An anecdote is told about a tribesman who, in the mid-twentieth century, was sprinting alongside a dirt road where auto traffic occasionally passed. "Want a lift?" yelled a motorist, as he geared down his low-slung red convertible.

The Native American didn't even break his stride, shook his head and shouted:

"No, thanks. I'm in a hurry."

Harrison Doyle, who for years lived among the Native Americans near Needles, California, on the Arizona state line, has many cherished memories of these times. As a youth he often ran races with young tribesmen.

Reason for Doyle's Defeats

Usually he would break in front of the group. However, after a few hundred yards, they all passed him. After about a mile, winded and exhausted, he fell far behind.

He asked his competitors how they were able to beat him every time. They cast knowing glances at one another, laughed, but refused to answer.

No matter how much he pleaded, the Native Americans never revealed their secret. Frustrated and determined to find the answer, Doyle carefully observed his competitors during entire days. Eventually he noted that on most mornings they would take seeds from pouches attached to their waistbands and chew on them.

He observed them gathering the seeds from tall, many-branched plants that grew wild near the edge of the reservation.

Clyde Hogan, of Paso Robles, California, a man who had spent much time with Doyle and interviewed him in-depth, told me:

"They turned out to be chia seeds. Harrison Doyle began chewing on them each morning, or soaking them in water for thirty minutes to an hour and drinking the mucilaginous product. At first he noticed little change in energy and endurance. However, after about six weeks, he experienced a big difference.

"Then he challenged the Native Americans to a long race. This time he stayed even with them and, before the finish line, surged ahead and won. Rather than feel disgruntled, the young braves just laughed. They knew Doyle had discovered their secret."[2]

Reminiscences

Doyle remembered a common sight: tribesmen filling pouches with chia seeds (often the only food taken, along with a gourd with water), strapping on a backpack, and running for days, covering 300 rugged miles along the Mojave Trail from Needles through the Cajon Pass to the California coast. There they traded blue and green stones (malachite copper and turquoise), chips of flint or obsidian lava, arrowheads, and sometimes ochre paint.

Among many tribes it was common for men to eat a tablespoon of chia before spending a day hunting for game.

A story is told of young, chia-fed Apache braves, stationed long distances apart, chasing after a deer for extended periods of time. Outdistanced at the start, they showed amazing endurance and energy in the pursuit. Finally the deer, became exhausted and was easy prey. Then they carried the animal for miles back to the village, showing no signs of overfatigue.

This legend challenged my ability to believe, but it was verified by Clyde Hogan, with whom Harrison Doyle discussed the subject. Doyle was an eye witness to several such hunts.

The motion picture *The Last of the Mohicans* opens with braves chasing down a deer, as described by Hogan.

Clyde Hogan also relates that running to a distant destination for hours, even days, was boring, so various Indian tribes occasionally amused themselves by taking part in a competitive game. Several hours after eating a tablespoon of chia, they would run nonstop at top speed, each one kicking a fur object stuffed with weeds, their equivalent of a ball. The purpose was to be the first to kick their "ball" across an agreed-upon finish line.

"Often their goal was twenty to twenty-five miles away," Hogan told me. "Such a competition took even more skill than that of a soccer player, because the objects kicked were anything but round, and required the endurance of a marathon runner. Even today's well-trained athletes might have dropped from exhaustion well before the finish line, but invariably all the braves completed the run, thanks to chia seed and the fear of losing face."

California coastal Native Americans often shared chia seed with Spanish missionary priests—among them, Father Junipero Serra—who, with a large party, journeyed by foot throughout the state, establishing missions. Chia gave them surprising strength and endurance.

Some ate chia seed that had been roasted and then ground, others made a refreshing drink from pure well or spring water, chia seed, a dash of lemon, and raw honey.

An Unforgettable Character

Adolph Bulla was a hard-rock desert miner in his seventies who was legendary for his physical stamina. Some years ago he was the subject of a feature story in the *Los Angeles Times*. After reading it, Harrison Doyle drove out to Randsburg, California, to interview Bulla.

"It was indeed astonishing to find a hard-rock miner at that age drilling, blasting, mucking, and hauling for six sunup-to-sundown days a week," he told Bob Andersen. "Crediting his remarkable physical stamina to chia seed, which grew up and down hills near his home, Bulla generously presented me with some, explaining that he mixes a teaspoonful into hot-cake batter—sometimes a little more for an especially hard day—and this fortifies him for work *without another meal.*" And despite constant exposure to the burning, skin-aging desert sun, Bulla "looked and acted a good twenty years younger than his actual age," according to Doyle.

Doyle claims that numerous Native Americans were sustained by only a tablespoonful of chia and a gourd of water on a twenty-four-hour forced march.

Massacre Canyon

How essential chia was to the economy of Native Americans is accented in Harrison Doyle's story of Massacre Canyon. Centuries ago at the location of today's city of San Jacinto, California, there once thrived the Indian village of Ivah.

"The supply of chia in that valley was plentiful, and the people of Ivah were prosperous," Doyle stated. "Then came a year of scant rainfall. Chia failed to mature in the nearby valleys, but on the highlands near Ivah, there was a plentiful supply.

"Indians from Temeculah, where the crop had failed, invaded the Ivah highlands to gather seed, and were battled by the outnumbered Ivahs, protecting their food supply. During the conflict, the Ivahs were forced into a narrow ravine where, backs to the wall, they fought to the death.

"When settlers came to the area and heard the story, handed down by the descendants of the brave defenders of Ivah's chia, they named the place Massacre Canyon," Doyle told Bob Andersen.

CHAPTER 3

Natural Food: The Early Years

Much of my fascination for chia, and for all natural foods, grew from frequent meetings with the late Francis M. Pottenger, Jr., M.D., in the offices of his respiratory clinic in the sunny, high hills above Monrovia, California.

Dr. Pottenger had a fullback's solid build, a jaunty step, an almost permanent, warm smile, and a thick mop of salt-and-pepper hair. He was a pioneer alternative and preventive physician, whose prescriptions were almost always natural foods and supplements.

Testimony to his hundreds of miraculous cures lined the walls of his reception room and offices: "before and after" photos of patients. In the "before mode, usually after a long illness, some patients resembled living skeletons, with bones for arms and legs, washboard ribs, and gaunt faces. In the "after" mode, they looked like body-beautifuls who could conquer the world. Some did. When I congratulated Dr. Pottenger on his achievements, he said, "Give natural foods the credit."

Super Supplements

He recommended and himself used traditional nutritional supplement builder-uppers such as brewer's yeast, desiccated liver, frozen, raw beef liver (grated into tomato juice), blackstrap molasses, a rice-bran-based vitamin B-complex, wheat germ oil, and whole-grain cereals, as well as fresh, organically grown fruits and vegetables and certified raw milk. He mentioned chia seed as a product to add to his health-restoring arsenal, regretting that it was not always available in nutrition centers.

That was where I first learned about chia. When I mentioned wanting to write and edit in the field of health and nutrition, Dr. Pottenger recommended that I read every health and nutrition article and book and hear every lecture by then leaders such as Adelle Davis, Carlton Fredericks, Lelord Kordel, Gaylord Hauser, W. Coda Martin, M.D., Joseph Risser, M.D., Beatrice Trum Hunter, Gladys Lindbergh, and Paul Bragg.

I did that and also launched a health publication, *Food-Wise*, distributed in health food stores throughout California. I was fortunate to have the contents of *Food-Wise* reviewed for accuracy by W. Coda Martin, M.D., one of the nation's most knowledgeable, nutrition-oriented physicians and a vigorous advocate of chia seed. Dr. Martin acted as health advisor to motion picture personality Gloria Swanson, noted for her enduring youthfulness.

Sally Spreads the Word

Another of my early exposures to chia seed was through a health food store distributor for *Food-Wise*, Sally Zerfing, owner of Sally's Health Store in Newhall, California, on the edge of the Mojave Desert.

Periodically I made visits to proprietors or managers of stores distributing my publication, asking for suggestions for future articles. It was eleven o'clock in the morning, and Sally offered me what she called Sally's Vitality Bar, a raw food candy bar including a generous ingredient of chia. I munched the Vitality Bar and found it much more tasty than most health food candy.

After visiting several other stores, I drove back to my home in the foothills of Altadena at about six o'clock in the evening. My wife had dinner ready, but I wasn't hungry; I picked at my food.

"What did you have for lunch?" she asked.

"Actually I didn't eat lunch, only a health food candy bar given me by Sally Zerfing."

Then I realized it was Sally's Vitality Bar that had made me feel satiated for seven hours.

That excited me about chia seed. What an appetite depressant, I thought, ideal for people who want to lose weight!

Not only did Sally Zerfing ignite my interest in chia, she also fired up that of Keith A. Tucker, then the football and wrestling coach at the William S. Hart High School in Newhall.

Tucker's athletes began eating Sally's Vitality Bar and, when available, chia seed to add to their breakfast food or to whole-grain pancakes and waffles. Invariably their athletic performances improved.

In a magazine article, Tucker wrote that Sally's Vitality Bar "gives an energy pickup about thirty minutes after it is eaten."[1]

Paul Bragg's Fascinating Feats

Following Dr. Pottenger's advice, I attended many nutrition lectures, including one by pioneer nutritionist Paul Bragg, and learned more exciting facts about chia seed. Bragg referred to the legendary physical feats performed by chia seed eaters down through history and related the absorbing story of how he had been introduced to this fabulous seed.

"Early in this century, two friends and I decided to climb the rugged and uncharted San Jacinto mountain that towered

10,831 feet above the then small southern California desert community of Palm Springs.

"This is one of the world's most spectacular mountains, inasmuch as it is situated in flat desert country and goes straight up. In our packsacks was food for three days. Starting at dawn, we struggled up to the top just as the sun was setting on the western horizon.

"Too tired to do anything else, we ate our evening meal and then crawled into our sleeping bags. Early next morning, a tremendous thunderstorm broke over the mountains. It was like being pounded by a waterfall. Drenched, we quickly ran under an overhang of rocks.

"When the cloudburst subsided, we were upset to find that our packsacks of food had been washed down the mountainside—along with our trail maps and guiding compass. Our situation was desperate. It is not easy to go down a mountain—miles and miles of wilderness—with thick underbrush and sheer dropoffs.

"Afraid of starving to death, we started downward on the wet, slippery, and rocky terrain. Of course, the trail was washed out. Just when we thought we were making progress, we came to a cliff with a dropoff of several thousand feet and had to start all over again.

"A long day of hiking through the underbrush and stumbling over rocks exhausted us, especially because we hadn't eaten a morsel of food. We were thankful we had canteens of water. We slept under a big Ponderosa pine that night.

"Our next day was almost a duplicate of the previous one. So were the following three days. Discouraged, apprehensive, and exhausted on the morning of the sixth day without food, we found that we were back where we had started on the first day.

"While we tried to figure out what to do, an Indian of the Agua Caliente tribe appeared out of nowhere. He had a remarkable body—tall, lean, symmetrical—and he moved with such power that I was amazed. He carried a rifle, and there was a leather pack on his back. His bronze skin almost glowed. I judged him to be middle-aged.

"He spoke excellent English, telling us he had been on a nine-day hunting trip looking for a mountain goat. I wondered how he had fed himself during that period. He showed us. His leather pack contained seeds which he called chia. He had lived on several teaspoonsful daily. Seeing that we were lost and famished, he shared some with us.

"Within a short time, the three of us us felt a supercharge of energy. Never in my life had I experienced such a sharp change. I told the Indian that I was made a blood brother in the Cherokee Indian tribe and given the name Gischuch-wipall-Wullamallesohen, translated into Rays of the Sun, and the Healer.

"That was my introduction to chia seed and to its remarkable powers to invigorate a person. Equally remarkable was the fact that this Indian, a powerful specimen of manhood, was seventy-nine years old and lived mainly on chia seed.

"Our Indian friend didn't need a trail to lead us out of the mountain. That night we bathed in the hot mineral water pools on the Agua Caliente reservation near Palm Springs. Next day, our friend took us out into the desert and showed us where the chia plants grew wild. It took us hours to harvest about a half pound. However, it was worth it.

"That top-of-the-mountain experience was one of the most trying of my life, but I wouldn't have missed it for anything. From that time on, I made a point of going to the desert to gather chia seed or to buy it whenever it was available in health food stores.

"Although I had eaten chia seeds for some time and, as an athlete, had gained strength and stamina in the process, I wanted more evidence that chia was the reason for these gains. After all, I ate a number of great health foods. I remembered something from the Bible, a quotation from the Apostle Paul to the Thessalonians: 'Prove all things.'"

That was what Paul Bragg did. The test came about almost by accident. In a chat with a group of young men and women athletes at his athletic club, he checked each person to find out which foods gave them the most energy, vitality, and endurance for winning performances.

Responses ranged from wheat germ, wheat germ oil, brewer's yeast, desiccated liver, blackstrap molasses, royal jelly and soy foods, to individual supplements such as vitamin C, vitamin B-complex, magnesium, and mineral complexes.

Chia Seed Put to the Test

"Then my turn came," said Bragg. "I quickly told the group I seemed to get my greatest go power from chia seed, which has been my old standby for energy for years—just as it has been for various American Indian tribes. Inasmuch as I was considered more or less a guru of the group, one of the young men said, 'Paul, why don't we test chia seed on some weekend?'"

There was almost unanimous agreement, and Paul Bragg structured the experiment, actually a competition—a grueling test of endurance, a thirty-six-hour hike to the top of Mount Wilson and into its wilderness back country. He divided the volunteers into two groups. "Members of one group were to eat only chia seed during the climb, and the others were to eat whatever foods they wished."

"I took the chia-seed-eating young people—eight men and four women—and another fellow led the eat-as-you-wish group. On a sunny yet nippy morning we started out. We in the chia-eating group took in several teaspoons of chia seed in water as soon as we arose. During the entire outing, we chewed on chia seeds or took them in water.

"For the first few hours, there seemed to be no difference in our ability to climb. However, as the terrain got rougher and the slopes steeper, things changed. Our chia-eating group started to pull ahead of the others.

"Initially, we were ahead by a quarter of a mile, then a half mile, and soon there was more than a mile between our group and the other. As we munched on the chia seeds, we negotiated the rough upgrade almost effortlessly. No one felt tired or recommended that we rest. Actually, we appeared to gain momentum as we covered the miles."

Soon Bragg's group was on the home stretch toward the agreed-upon goal. At the end, everyone in his group appeared recharged and even ready to go farther. Out of the other group of twelve, only five finished—three men and two women—and they dragged in four hours and twenty-seven minutes after Paul Bragg's chia-eating group.

Dramatic Results

All of them were exhausted, their faces drawn and their feet dragging. They were almost too played out even to talk. None of them needed to be convinced that chia spelled the difference between winning and losing the Mount Wilson competition.

"Even before that contest, I suspected that chia seeds were one of the greatest foods I had discovered to help refuel my body engine," Bragg told us. "Our Mount Wilson competition convinced me of that fact.

"Inasmuch as I have lived my life in California as a great admirer of the American Indian, I learned the true value of chia seeds. Night after night, for many, many years, I have added a teaspoonful of chia seeds to a glass of water to soak, ready for me to drink upon rising in the morning. Chia is a wonder—an old-fashioned marvel in a modern world. It has charged me up with extra drive that no other food has."

Zealous about Chia Seed

Almost evangelical in his desire for everybody to try chia, Paul Bragg finished his talk by saying,

"The Indians depended on chia seed to give them extra go power. Now nutrition-minded people in various parts of the country are using chia seeds in many different ways. As I discuss the subject with people after my lectures, I find they are delighted with the additional energy and endurance they receive from chia seed. In this age of the rat race, it is comforting to know that sound nutrition can furnish that extra fuel to help us maintain the required terrific pace."

Bragg then expressed thankfulness for seeds in general and chia in particular, also recommending sunflower seeds, pumpkin seeds, raw wheat germ, brewer's yeast, and other health-giving and energy-providing natural foods. Then he challenged us in the audience:

"Test chia for yourself to determine it's nutritional worth— not necessarily on a rugged, thirty-six-hour mountain hike. See if adding chia seeds to your diet doesn't give you that extra charge of energy that will help you to finish your days in high gear. Chia is for everyone. No age limits. See for yourself!"[2]

My Turn for a Test

I wanted to see for myself. However, no nearby health food store stocked chia seed. Then, in time, I got busy writing and editing, and I forgot about chia, Sally Zerfing's Vitality Bar, and the experiences with chia seed of Keith A. Tucker, Paul Bragg, and Native Americans.

However, when I met Bob Andersen, this wealth of information flooded back to me, and I found long-forgotten notes I had taken about chia. Bob gave me a liberal supply of chia seed samples.

One Friday evening I soaked a tablespoon of chia seed in a glass of spring water. On the following morning, at about 8:30, I asked my wife, Joan, to add the now-gelatinous and swollen volume of chia to the batter for whole-grain pancakes.

Before we each ate three large pancakes with butter and maple syrup, we had a small bowl of fresh fruit: peaches, pears, apples, and bananas. Then we both went to our home-office suites, Joan to compose music on her computer, and I to start work on a magazine article.

A Wow Experience

We both became so deeply involved in our projects that we lost awareness of time. However, no matter how exciting the work I'm doing, I usually hear my inner alarm clock at about noon, telling me it's time to raise my blood sugar level.

However, I felt not the least energy letdown and, as I wrote with my word processor, I happened to look at my wristwatch and was amazed to find that it was 2:30 in the afternoon—six hours from when we had eaten, and I was only mildly hungry. Joan reported the same reaction!

Wow!

CHAPTER 4

Chia Folk Medicine

Above and beyond its richness in essential nutrients, chia seed has been valued for its medicinal qualities since the beginning of recorded history. Today's chia seed eaters may want to know the many ways that the Aztecs, Mayas, Tehuantapecs, Tarahumaras, and other Native Americans used it to prevent and manage physical ailments.

For very good reasons, botanists classified chia as a sage, a member of the mint family. The sages are called *Salvias,* derived from the Latin "salvere," meaning "to save" or "salvage." This is exactly what legends indicate that chia seed did for the Aztecs and Native Americans who were not well.

Harrison Doyle, a virtual magnet for stories from Native Americans about chia, tells of its amazing revival power. A prospector, prostrate near a desert water hole, is about to die.

An old Indian brave comes by, realizes what is about to happen, takes a handful of chia from a pouch at his waist, stirs the seeds in water in a gourd until they are mush and slowly feeds it to the dying man. The mush stays down, and the next morning the prospector is back on his feet, his will to live and life restored.[1]

For Colds and Childbirth

When Native Americans had colds and sore throats, they soaked chia seed in water overnight and then swallowed the resulting gelatinous mass. This or oil pressed from chia seeds served as an emollient, something that soothed inflamed mucus membranes, including bronchial membranes, or irritated skin.

Neither Harrison Doyle nor tribal lore mentions premenstrual syndrome (PMS). Perhaps it would be an oversimplification to imply that PMS was rare among Indian women due to their rich intake of omega-3 oil in chia seed.

However, many studies show that omega-3 fatty acids are helpful in lessening symptoms of PMS—cramps, nervousness, breast-swelling, bloating, or crying jags—and, in some cases, preventing them.

To ease childbirth, Native American women were usually fed additional chia seed. By eating more of it regularly while pregnant, they assured their babies great health benefits.

Now Dr. Morton Walker, a leading health writer, reports a rationale for this. Omega-3 and omega-6 essential fatty acids, such as those in chia seed, fed to pregnant women, help to assure the fetus normal development of brain, central nervous system, and retina, the part of the eye that receives the image.[2]

Experiments with rhesus monkeys showed that if the pregnant female doesn't take in sufficient DHA, a key ingredient in omega-3 oil, the infant will also be deficient, reports Dr. Walker.

This finding prompted researchers at the Oregon Health Sciences University (Portland) and at the Instituto de Nutricion y Technologia de los Alimentos at the University of Chile (Santiago) to see if these findings also apply to pregnant human beings and their fetuses.[3]

Put to the Test

Thirty-one healthy, pregnant women volunteered for the Oregon study. Fifteen received a nine-week dietary supplement of omega-3 EFAs, starting with their twenty-sixth week up to the thirty-fifth week. (The supplement was derived from skinless, boneless sardines and fish oils such as cod liver oils.) Omega-3 from fish oils is similar to that derived from seeds such as chia and other plants. However, the former costs more.

A second group of sixteen served as controls. In the supplemented pregnant women, omega-3 in their red blood cells rose from 4.69 percent of total fatty acids to 7.15 percent at the end of the supplementation. Benefits of supplementation to mothers were passed on to their infants. Omega-3 in the red blood cells of supplemented mothers measured at 7.92 percent of total fatty acids, compared with only 5.86 percent for mothers of control infants.

A Verifying Study

Results of the Santiago experiment were similar. Omega-3-deficient mothers gave birth to infants with negatively altered brain and retinal functions.

Dr. Walker quoted the Santiago researcher as follows:

"Our results to date indicate that omega-3 fatty acids are required for optimal retinal and brain development in human infants and, thus, should be considered essential nutrients for infant nutrition."

Without these nutrients infants won't be able to catalyze the breakdown of fatty acids and won't be able to readily detoxify certain molecules that are parts of pollutants, including environmental cancer-causatives, he indicates.

Based on these studies, Dr. Walker writes:

"One reason that cancer more frequently affects people in industrialized Western countries is that they ingest insufficient amounts of essential fatty acids, especially DHA," (a substance that the body derives from omega-3).

Essential for Fetuses and Newborns

Ricardo Uauy, M.D., Ph.D, from the University of Chile, states: "For developing fetuses and newborns, essential fatty acids (with omega-3 being vital among them) are the second most important structural component in the body after proteins, and are the most critical ingredients of the brain."

From these studies, Dr. Walker concludes that, for the sake of their fetuses and newborns-to-be, pregnant women should supplement their diets with DHA and related essential fatty acids.

Dr. Jay Lombard, a board-certified neurologist, and nutritionist Carl Germano offer some fascinating information on the need for omega-3 fatty acids for the brain in their book *The Brain Wellness Plan.*[4]

Brain Benefits

The DHA in omega-3 oil is a major structural fatty acid in the gray matter of the brain, they write. It does many important things in the brain. As an antioxidant it protects brain cells from free radicals. These are molecular muggers that attack adjacent molecules and injure them and can start a chain reaction of destruction.

DHA stimulates the immune system and helps to keep the brain healthy and functioning at peak potential. It "promotes communication between brain cells by allowing synapses (contact points where nerve impulses pass from one cell to another) to remain soft and functional."[4]

Lombard and Germano claim that lower amounts of omega-3 in infant formulas, compared with that in breast milk, led to lower intelligence in babies who were fed these formulas. Once the World Health Organization spread the word that DHA is a *must* for normal brain development, most companies making infant formulas now add DHA to them. (Be sure to check ingredients!)

DHA teams with another nutrient, phosphatidylserine, to keep cell membranes fluid. This is necessary for them to take in oxygen and food and to discharge wastes. It is also essential for cells to "speak" to one another by sending chemical messengers back and forth, according to Lombard and Germano.

Defense Against Alzheimer's Disease

More than likely, DHA defends the brain against Alzheimer's disease, they state. The major phospholipid ingredient of cell membranes that surround neurons in the brain is DHA. The brain contains various fats. Even a seemingly trivial amount of change in the lipid structure influences the way in which cell membranes pass neurotransmitters in and out.

"Many researchers believe that changes in the composition and metabolism of fatty acids like DHA may contribute to Alzheimer's disease," write Lombard and Germano. "In one major Swedish study, investigators demonstrated that the brain content of Alzheimer's patients was *significantly* (accentuation mine) less than the levels in the brains of control patients."[5]

In a study of essential fatty acids, Dr. Michael T. Murray drives home the point that omega-3 oil from flax seed or other grasses, grains, or seeds costs only one-sixth that of omega-3 oil from seafood sources.[6]

What he doesn't say is that flax seed is not actually a food. It has to be treated by several chemical processes in order for its oil to be used for human consumption. Chia seed doesn't.

A Better Balance of Omegas

Dr. Murray states that the intake of omega-6 far exceeds that of omega-3 and may upset the natural balance of these oils.

"Based on substantial evidence, it is estimated that the level of omega-6 oil in body tissues of most Americans is twenty times the level of omega-3. Most experts in fatty acid nutrition believe the optimum ratio of omega-6 to omega-3 is between three to one and four to one."

Therefore, supplementing the omega-3 oils results in a significant improvement in how the body works, because of far-reaching effects of hormone-like prostaglandin substances produced by omega-3 oils.

Some conditions that improved by supplementing the diet with omega-3 oils include high cholesterol levels, prevention of strokes and heart attacks, angina, high blood pressure, rheumatoid arthritis, multiple sclerosis, psoriasis and eczema, and cancer (prevention and treatment), states Dr. Murray.

Less Omega-6 and More Omega-3

In a special report, "Eating Fat, Then and Now," Mary Clarke, Ph.D., of Nutrition Education at Kansas State University, writes that the ratio between omega-6 and omega-3 up until this century had been one to one.[7]

Citing a study, "Dietary Polyunsaturated Fatty Acids and Depression," by Hibbeln and Salem, in the *American Journal of Clinical Nutrition*, 62 (1): 1–9, July 1995, she writes:

"When margarines made from vegetable oils became popular, this ratio changed so that omega-6s now far outnumber omega-3s by ratios from ten to one to as high as twenty-five to one. Accumulating evidence suggests that this change is an important factor in our high incidence of coronary heart disease and some other chronic diseases."

Dr. Clarke cites another possible problem with the lopsided ratio of omega-6 to omega-3 in the American diet: the rising rate of depression.

"No one is saying that the fat or oil you eat is the reason for more depression, because depression is the result of many factors, including genetics and environment. What researchers are suggesting is that certain individuals may become depressed more easily because of a long-standing imbalance in the kinds of unsaturated fats and oils they eat. Perhaps more omega-3s and fewer omega-6s might help."

Another authority on the omega fatty acids, William Lands, Ph.D., of the National Institute on Alcohol Abuse and Alcoholism, told an American Heart Association conference on omega-3 fatty acids something similar: the excessive intake of omega-6 in salad oils, mayonnaise, and margarine causes a buildup in human beings that suppresses and conceals the many benefits from omega-3 fatty acids.[8]

"You can't do overnight studies on omega-3 when there's a three-year supply of omega-6 staring you right back in the eyes," he said. It is worth noting that chia seeds contain a near sixty-to-forty ratio of omega-3s to omega-6s—a favorable ratio created by nature.

Chia authority Robert Kleiman, of International Flora Technologies, of Apache Junction, Arizona, told me that "it has recently been substantiated that alpha-linolenic acid, present in chia seed, is an essential fatty acid. This means that we must eat food with this fatty acid in it, because we cannot synthesize it.

"Both soybean oil and canola oil contain less than ten percent of this fatty acid. Chia, on the other hand, has about sixty percent of its oil as alpha-linolenic acid, which is the highest among any commercial oils.

"In the body, this essential fatty acid is converted to eicosapentaenoic acid (EPA) and docosahexaenoic acid (DHA), two fatty acids also found in fish oils. These two acids have been credited for the lower incidence of heart disease found in Greenland Eskimos, even though they eat a high-fat diet derived from blubber and meat."[9]

More Benefits

Chia seeds present additional advantages.

"Other societies such as the Scandinavians and Japanese, which eat large amounts of fish, also have a lower incidence of heart disease," continued Kleiman. "DHA, besides helping to reduce heart disease, is found in the retina of infants' eyes and, in large amounts, in the brain tissue of rats, indicating a role in many body areas and functions.

"This is the most prevalent fatty acid produced from alpha-linolenic acid by the body. Chia seed offers greater alpha-linolenic acid concentrations than any other seed or grain. Although expensive dietary supplements containing EPA and DHA can be bought, the body will produce these acids from chia seed and its oil," concluded Kleiman.

In the paper "Essential Fatty Acids and Nutritional Disorders," biochemist Ralph Holman cites a case study showing the effectiveness of linolenic acid as compared with linoleic acid. (There is appreciably more linolenic acid than linoleic acid in chia.)

Unusual Case Study

A six-year-old girl was accidentally wounded in the abdomen by a gunshot and had to have damaged parts of her small bowel removed surgically. During hospitalization her supplementary dietary regimen included an emulsion rich in linoleic acid but low in linolenic acid.

"Within five months, she experienced episodes of numbness, paresthesia (tingling or creeping of the skin), weakness, inability to walk, leg pain, and blurred vision," writes Holman.

Analysis of her blood serum level revealed a significant deficiency of linolenic acid and a marginal deficiency of linoleic acid. When she was placed on a supplement with a dominance of linolenic acid, her symptoms disappeared over the next twelve weeks, showing that the linolenic acid deficiency had been corrected.

Validation that linolenic acid can help wound-healing from the inside out is shown by a rat study reported by Holman. Omega-3 from vegetable, grain, and seed sources proved to contribute to faster wound-healing than that from fish sources.[10]

More Chia Folk Medicine

LINOLENIC AND LINOLEIC ACID IN A POULTICE OF MUSH MADE from chia seed contributed to efficient wound healing for Native Americans. In addition to gelatinous chia seed, the poultice contained pure water, a teaspoon of sage honey, and a dash of lemon juice, observed Harrison Doyle.[1]

Pioneers learned from friendly Native Americans how to prepare the poultice to apply to gunshot wounds, infections, and skin irritations. The mush was heated, wrapped in a clean cloth or in clean plant leaves and applied and held on or lashed with leather thongs to swollen or sore areas. Infection was supposedly drawn out by this treatment.

Chia seed was eaten by Native Americans of the southwest for a wide range of unrelated ailments: upset stomach, body odor, prostate problems (yes, a small number of oldsters suffered from them), constipation, and overweight.

Suffering from upset stomach when nothing stays down, the Native Americans found that the same chia seed formula that worked for wound-healing would help if taken internally. It stayed down and cooled inflamed stomach membranes, Doyle told Bob Andersen.

For use as a deodorant, chia seed soaked in water overnight was made into a poultice that was placed in the armpits before the users went to sleep.

Tribal lore held that this cleansed the sweat glands. On the eve of a planned hunt, braves effectively deodorized their armpits, not for social acceptability but for an even more important reason: for keeping game from detecting a human odor and fleeing.

Prostate Problems

One of chia's legendary uses by elderly male Native Americans and pioneers was to relieve the need for frequent urination, incontinence, occasionally painful urination, and lower back pain related to prostate problems, explained Doyle.

In those days sufferers from these symptoms didn't know that their ailment was probably benign prostatic hyperplasia (BPH), enlargement of the prostate gland. However, they did know that a daily drink of a tablespoonful of chia seed (soaked in glass of water until gelatinous) for twenty to thirty consecutive days helped to lessen their problem—or even alleviate it.

Before offering a possible explanation for this, we should understand more about the prostate, a gland whose purpose is to secrete a milky white fluid to carry sperm cells out of the penis. The prostate surrounds the narrow neck of the bladder, the urethra, a flexible tube at the base of the penis. Urine is discharged through this tube.

With advancing age, the prostate usually enlarges. In a few cases, cancer causes enlargement. Either condition makes the prostate tighten like a vise, causing all sorts of urinary problems: difficulty starting to urinate, difficulty fully evacuating the bladder, or even completely blocking the flow, necessitating catheterization.

Can the Omegas Help?

Whatever reduces the enlarged prostate can often eliminate the uncomfortable symptoms of BPH. More than a half century ago, several studies revealed that prostate patients' prostatic and seminal fat levels were low and their ratios abnormal. However, researchers didn't immediately realize that supplementation with an essential fatty acid complex might help.

It was discovered in clinical tests that a daily teaspoon of the essential fatty acid linoleic acid (omega-6 oil), from which arachidonic acid is synthesized, and omega-3 oil improved many BPH patients. (Chia contains generous amounts of both linoleic and linolenic acid.)

Then, too, in an uncontrolled study, nineteen out of nineteen patients, after several weeks on these essential fatty acids, showed a decline in residual urine and improved ability to empty the bladder. Twelve of the nineteen were able to empty their bladders completely.[2]

Attention Doctors and Patients!

A disease of modern civilization, multiple sclerosis (MS), appears to respond to a good intake of both omega-3 fatty acids, DHA and EPA. Like rheumatoid arthritis and lupus erythematosus, MS is an autoimmune disease. This means that the immune system attacks healthy body tissues—in this instance, the myelin sheaths that protect nerves, like insulation protects an electric wire.

Then inflammation attacks the naked nerves, making them transmit faulty signals. Symptoms can vary depending upon the areas of myelin sheath damage: bladder and bowel ailments, blurred or double vision, breathing difficulty, incontinence, impotence, numbness, muscle spasms, paralysis, skin ulcers, and urinary tract infections.

Linoleic and linolenic acids, essential fatty acids, are shown to help control symptoms of MS and, in some instances, to reverse them. EFAs are converted into prostaglandins, substances that perform short-term, hormonelike actions, such as controlling blood pressure and smooth muscle contractions.

Linolenic acid has been used for more than a half century in Europe to manage MS. An article in *Spectrum News* states that "Flax seed oil contains from fifty to sixty percent linolenic acid and is also important in treating MS." Chia oil contains slightly more: 60.8 percent.[3]

Individuals who eat a high percentage of saturated fats and cholesterol and drink alcohol heavily usually increase the severity of their MS symptoms.

A study of 146 MS patients revealed that, in patients on a low-fat diet for an average of seventeen years, this disease progressed far less rapidly than in those on a high-fat diet. Further, symptoms of the first group were less frequent and severe than those in the latter group.[4]

European alternative doctors who placed their MS patients on a low-fat diet *and* supplemented them with essential fatty acids as well as vitamins and minerals, reported the greatest success with MS patients.[5]

Weight Problems

Another serious physical condition, one that troubles many women and men, is overweight. In decades of living near and with various Native Americans tribes and observing thousands of individuals, Harrison Doyle maintained that he never saw an obese person who ate chia seed regularly. Presumably this is because chia seeds in water swell by seven times and, in the stomach, give a feeling of complete satiation.

Mixed with orange juice, the gel-like seeds make a nutritious breakfast and can help to control excess weight. "Users report that a glass full of orange juice with a teaspoon of pre-soaked chia seeds leaves one feeling full and without hunger until noon," Harrison Doyle told me.

Unlike crash diets consisting of a high volume of low-calorie, low-nutrition food or fluids in the stomach to produce a feeling of fullness, chia seed brings satiation and nutritional richness with few calories. Some individuals I know use the water-dissolved gelatin from chia seed as a supplement to one or more meals and invariably slash their daily intake of calories, while still obtaining essential nutrients.

Constipation

The inability to evacuate the bowels regularly was rarely a problem for native Americans, because they were physically active, drank sufficient water, and usually took in ample fiber in foods. The aged and otherwise sedentary men and women solved the irregularity problem with a daily teaspoon of chia seed dissolved in water, Doyle said.

Chia seed supplies fiber in two forms: insoluble (won't dissolve in water) from its outer coat and soluble (will dissolve in water) from the inner ingredients.

The first type, containing cellulose and lignin, helps to prevent or ease constipation. The second type has been found helpful in lowering cholesterol and managing diabetes.

Dangers of Constipation

The word "constipation" comes from a Latin phrase *con stipari,* which means "crammed together," exactly the state of waste matter in the colon of those having difficulty becoming regular. This Latin meaning illustrates vividly the danger of waste matter lingering too long in the lower colon. Toxins from foods and the environment are eliminated in two major ways—in solid waste matter and in the urine.

Experiments of Dr. Robert Bruce, director of the Toronto Branch of the Ludwig Cancer Research Institute, show that long-contained solid wastes putrefy, and the longer they press against the sensitive bowel membrane, the greater the threat of colon cancer, a scourge second only to lung cancer.[6]

Warnings about constipation and its more serious physical complications have been sounded for almost two hundred years and little heeded.

Way back in the early 1800s Sylvester Graham (after whom graham flour and the graham cracker were named) preached the need to eat only bakery products made from whole-grain flours. Already millers were removing the bran and germ from grains, turning out increasing tonnage of white flour.

Few people listened. Then in the 1930s Dr. C.R. Cowgill, a Yale University physiology professor, revealed with experiments that fiber—not some mysterious ingredient—helped keep bowel movements normal. Very few people listened.

In the 1940s Dr. Alexander Walker, a South African biochemist, dramatically revealed the disease-prevention and health benefits from fiber. When black natives moved from rural areas, where fiber-containing foods were plentiful, to large cities, where refined foods were low-cost, popular, and plentiful, their incidence of colon diseases soared. Still, few people listened. After all, the drug stores were full of laxatives.

People Listened to Burkitt

Only when a surgeon named Denis Burkitt, a medical missionary from Uganda, returned to England and announced his discovery that dietary fiber is essential to regularity, did an appreciable part of the world's population began to pay attention.

Natives of Uganda rarely were hospitalized for constipation, colon cancer, or heart disease. Their diets were rich in bowel-moving, fibrous plant foods. On the other hand, English residents of Uganda, who ate breads made with refined, white flour and much meat, suffered constipation, colon cancer, and heart disease.

Many millions throughout the world heeded Dr. Burkitt's announcement, and a marked trend toward natural, unrefined foods began.

However, most people in the United States are still hung up on processed, refined, fiber-stripped, preservative-containing, fat-laden junk foods. Americans eat only one-fifth as much fiber as they did a hundred years ago.

Although a conservative U.S. Surgeon General urged individuals to take in at least thirty-five grams of fiber daily, the average person consumes only nine to twelve grams daily. Why so little? Mainly because typical American diets accent meat, poultry, dairy products, and processed foods. Further, they avoid or minimize fresh fruit and vegetables, so-called "rabbit food."

Soluble fiber, like that derived from soaked chia seeds, helps to prevent many serious medical conditions.

The Spiller Recommendation

Gene A. Spiller, D.Sc. and Ph.D., director of the Health Research and Studies Center in Los Altos, California, writes that his organization achieved the following results by increasing the amount of soluble fiber in the diets of individuals with high cholesterol: LDL cholesterol (the bad type) went down and HDL (the good type) stayed the same, making the relationship of the two more favorable for preventing cardiovascular complications.[7]

A Stanford University study revealed a finding similar to that of Spiller. Researchers recommended that otherwise healthy men and women with modestly elevated cholesterol (an average of 200) take fifteen grams daily of water-soluble fiber made from guar gum, locust bean gum, psyllium husks, and pectin. Within four weeks the average cholesterol of volunteers dropped by 8.3 percent and—of even greater significance—the LDL dropped by 12.4 percent!

Dr. Spiller adds that high fiber diets can help in managing diabetes.

"The absorption of sugar from the intestines is modified by fiber, and fiber might help to prevent the overweight tendency closely linked to adult diabetes."[8]

There's much more about the relation of high-fiber, natural-food diets to diabetes prevention in Chapters Seven and Eight.

A generation ago, Victor L. Frank, M.D., of Pasadena, California, was one of the few medical doctors to recommend daily use of chia to all his patients, for constipation, digestive disorders, lack of energy and stamina, and tired heart.

It is reported that he urged a local industrial company to try an experiment and request that its employees try chia on a daily basis. The company owner agreed. Management reported that, among employees who went along with the experiment, there was a production increase of about twenty percent in piece work.[9]

CHAPTER 6

The Inside Story

IF CHIA SEED IS SO HEALTHFUL, WHY IS SO LITTLE KNOWN about it?

First, it was at its height of popularity in cultures that no longer exist as such—the Aztecs, the Mayas, and the Tehuantapecs. Along with beans, corn, and amaranth, chia was a favorite food.

The Spanish invaders wantonly destroyed many cultural artifacts of the Aztecs and Mayas, often because their practices and customs went against the tenets of the Spaniards' religion and also to demonstrate their dominance.

Although the domestication of chia spread throughout Mexico, the practice of cultivating it in great abundance did not. Natives of what is now the southwestern United States gathered, processed, and ate chia that grew wild. These early Americans were more hunters than food growers.

Chia Domestication

Four agricultural researchers convinced the National Science Foundation to fund a research project to determine the feasibility of domesticating chia: H.E. Gentry, of Botanical Research & Development Corp., of Scottsdale, Arizona; R.L. Whistler, of Whistler Center for Carbohydrate Research, Purdue University, West Lafayette, Indiana; Marc Mittleman, Amerind Agrotech Laboratories; and P.R. McCrohan, Gentry Experimental Farms, Murrietta, California.

These men experimented for years with how to turn wild chia into a dependable domesticated crop and reported their progress to the National Science Foundation. This is an excerpt from what they wrote:

"In our endeavor, we will be on the frontier of a special branch of agricultural science. Our objective will be to select plants that will become a new crop for the United States Southwest.

"If successful, we can achieve obvious benefits: diversifying agriculture with a new industry; increasing the health of people who exercise too little and eat too much; conserving water by substituting water-economical chia for water-hogging crops, such as cotton and alfalfa.... We will also correct the agricultural neglect of these useful plants which has gone on for a century."

Driving Without a Map

Admitting that the domestication of foreign and wild plants is difficult and time-consuming, they stated: "Our ancestors have domesticated far more plants than we have, but they required centuries of time and were really hungry. There is no written guide to growing the various chias, not even in Mexico.

"We can only learn the cultural requirements of these little-known plants by working and living with them season by season and year by year. We can meet the challenge with our experience as trained specialists with other plants.

"The product of the chias are small seeds which have been eaten for centuries by native North Americans.... Chemists of the Northern Regional Research Center made several analyses of seeds of *Hyptia suaveolens* and *Salvia columbariae* (two kinds of chia). M.O. Bagby, of that institution, writes of *H. suaveolens:*

"Their oil contents were 22.8, 13.3, and 15.3 percent. The fatty acid composition of the seed oils was somewhat like that of a high linoleic safflower oil: 70 percent. It is also claimed that the seeds are an excellent dietary food in helping to control excess weight."[1]

Richest in Healthful Oil

This biochemical report reveals chia seed oil's high-quality unsaturated fatty acids. Degree of unsaturation is shown by what is called "the iodine number." Chia seed oil is among the highest known, at 197.[2]

One analytical report states, "With respect to polyunsaturated fatty acids (PUFAs), chia ranks at the top in comparison to other oil seeds with high linoleic and linolenic acids."

A little-known champion among polyunsaturates, chia seed oil rates a top score by far—81.2, followed by its closest competitors—safflower oil, with a 75, and sunflower oil with a 67.[3]

Oil of the chia seed has been found extremely high in the polyunsaturated fatty acid linolenic acid (omega-3) oil: 60.8 percent. This is highly significant for your and my good health and well-being.[4]

PUFAs and the Heart

To lessen the risk of heart disease, the American Heart Association, over the last generation, has urged raising the intake of PUFAs and reducing the intake of saturated fats.

The most important PUFA, linoleic acid is richly present in chia oil. However, the business-as-usual way of processing may convert linoleic acid from its active *cis* form to its inactive *trans* form. In other words, processing may cancel its essential fatty acid (EFA) effectiveness.

Most experts agree that only PUFAs with essential fatty acid effectiveness are helpful in preventing heart disease. What is so significant about EFAs? A quick look at their history will offer a resounding answer to that question.

Striking Discoveries

A husband-and-wife research team, George and Mildred Burr at the University of Minnesota, discovered EFAs in 1929. Even more important, they found that, without EFAs in their diets, animals showed an amazing range of symptoms: poor and slow growth, failure to reproduce, falling hair, and a host of unsightly skin ailments.

First the skin became scaly, then it broke out into a rash, with lesions resembling those of eczema. The animals developed numerous blood clots, hemorrhages, wounds that refused to heal, and showed an amazing susceptibility to infections.[5]

Researcher David Horrobin, Ph.D., a world authority on PUFAs, reports in an article, "Gamma-Linolenic Acid In Medicine," that, in a severe deficiency of EFAs, the skin throughout the body became porous, leaking water and leading to a perilous loss of body fluids. Animals drank copious amounts of water, but this didn't prevent kidney damage and death.[6]

What Dr. Horrobin Learned

Why did these unforeseen conditions arise? Because EFAs play two vital roles in every organ of the body. Here is how Dr. Horrobin explains it:

"The EFAs are part of the structure of every single tissue in the body, especially the brain, where very large amounts of EFA are found. The EFAs are major components of all cell membranes within the body. Without normal amounts of EFAs in the membranes, membranes become stiff and unable to function properly.

"The EFAs can give rise to very short-lived substances called prostaglandins (PGs). PGs play a role in regulating second-by-second function of every part of the body. Each organ produces its own PGs; these PGs are made from the EFAs stored in the organ, perform their functions, and then are almost instantly destroyed so that they cannot influence what is happening in other organs. Each organ, therefore, has its own PGs which perform their specific tasks."

Linolenic acid translates into alpha-linolenic acid (ALA), which converts to EPA and DHA, necessary for the formation of certain prostaglandins.

A Biochemical Obstacle Course

Another conversion is necessary—that of linoleic acid. Although on average we take in about five to fifteen grams of linoleic acid each day, this doesn't guarantee that linoleic acid will become transformed into the highly desirable gamma-linolenic acid (GLA).

Let's consider an analogy. Beta carotene cannot be transformed into vitamin A unless it goes through certain chemical changes in the liver, and the liver must be functioning normally for this to happen.

There's a towering problem with linoleic acid. Young children can readily convert it into gamma-linolenic acid. Adults can't. Although ninety-nine percent of linoleic acid cannot be converted into GLA, linoleic acid remains a reliable source of energy—one of the reasons chia seems such a nutritional powerhouse.

There are several major reasons why linoleic acid isn't converted to GLA: (1) high blood cholesterol levels; (2) too much saturated fat and harmful trans-fatty acids from eating processed junk foods; (3) high amounts of released adrenalin due to over-stress; (4) alcohol in the system, inasmuch as ten percent of calories consumed by North Americans come from alcohol; (5) diabetes; (6) atopy.[7]

What is atopy?

Here is Dr. Horrobin's explanation:

"Atopy is an inherited susceptibility to certain diseases such as eczema, asthma, and allergic rhinitis. It is the susceptibility rather than the actual illness which is inherited. It is common to find families where one member has asthma, another rhinitis, and where some unfortunates have two or even three conditions.... About one person in five or six is atopic.... Over seventy percent of women with menstrual syndrome and over seventy percent of hyperactive children come from atopic families."

Difficulty in metabolizing linoleic acid in atopic eczema was first demonstrated in 1957 by Arild Hansen, a pediatrician from the University of Minnesota, writes Dr. Horrobin. This work lay almost unknown for over forty years until it was rediscovered and confirmed by modern techniques. Clearly, people with atopy have a defect in their ability to convert linoleic acid into gamma-linolenic acid.[8]

In atopic conditions, victims lack a certain enzyme needed to perform the conversion. Human milk is one of the few foods containing gamma-linolenic acid. Some authorities state that breast-fed babies from healthy mothers are usually spared any atopic conditions.

Evening primrose oil and oil from borage and black currant seeds have been the only substantial supplemental source for adults to take in sufficient GLA.

GLA: A Winner

Some linoleic acid from chia seeds may make it through the body's complex conversion process to become GLA. Gamma-linolenic acid has been shown by many double-blind studies to improve atopic conditions such as eczema, to lower blood cholesterol levels, to block some of the ill effects of alcoholism, to relieve dry eye syndrome, and to minimize or eliminate hyperactivity (attention deficit disorders).

One of the most difficult skin disorders to clear up by orthodox medical treatment is psoriasis—bright red outbreaks of the skin, laced with silvery scales. These red patches can erupt on any part of the body but seem to prefer the arms, legs, palms of the hands, elbows, knees, buttocks, and scalp.

Sometimes thyroid supplementation helps make these lesions diminish or disappear, as does a gluten-free diet or avoidance of common food allergens such as corn, citrus fruits, nuts, milk and acid beverages—coffee and soft drinks—and acid-containing pineapple or tomatoes.

S.S. Bleehan, M.D., a professor of dermatology at the Royal Hallamshire Hospital, Sheffield, England, found still another way. He gave psoriasis patients ten omega-3 capsules daily for twelve weeks. The treatment partially alleviated their itching and reduced their redness and scaling. Chia seeds are one of the richest botanical sources of omega-3 oil.[9]

Many Merits of Chia Seed Oil

Although many polyunsaturated oils on store shelves tend to lose their nutritional value due to rapid oxidation, this is not true of chia seed oil. A research team found that chia oil contains the antioxidants chlorogenic and caffeic acids, which, to some extent, retard the rate of oxidation.[10]

Chia seed is twenty percent protein on a dry weight basis, writes James Brown, president of International Flora Technologies, Ltd., of Apache Junction, Arizona.

"Chia seed contains almost two times the protein of other grains, three to ten times the oil of other grains (an omega-3 oil) and as much or more dietary fiber compared to other grains. Chia is simply one of the most nutritious grains cultivated by man."[11]

Brown's report states that chia is rich in mucopolysaccharides and that this "viscous mucopolysaccharide" imparts some desirable qualities to the seed so it can be eaten whole, in cakes, or used in beverages.

An A Grade for B Vitamins and Calcium

Perhaps another of the secrets to chia's contribution to high energy and endurance is its content of B vitamins. As little as one ounce of chia seed was found to contain the following percentages of key B vitamins in relation to the RDA: two percent of B-2 (riboflavin); thirteen percent of niacin, and twenty-nine percent of thiamin—the latter a sparkplug vitamin for metabolizing carbohydrates for energy.[12]

Some biochemists say that the ratio of B vitamins to one another is almost as important as high individual amounts. Chia has been found to contain at least trace amounts of all of the major fractions of the vitamin B family.

Chia seed contains such a whopping amount of calcium that even researchers doing the chemical analysis were amazed and tested samples several times before believing their findings.

In roughly two ounces of chia seed (100 grams) there were 600 milligrams of calcium, contrasted with 120 milligrams in 100 grams of milk—five times as much, writes James Brown.[13] This makes chia seed a phenomenal source of calcium over milk for those who are lactose intolerant.

High in Boron Content

Chia also boasts the critically needed trace mineral boron, thought to be present only in fruits, vegetables, almonds, dates, unprocessed honey, peanuts, prunes, raisins, and soybeans.[14]

Several studies show that boron is severely depleted or totally absent from soils in various parts of the United States—the Atlantic coastal plain, the northwest Pacific and the state of Wisconsin. One authority states that fifty million acres of U.S. croplands require the addition of boron to their soil and only twenty-five percent of this land is getting it.[15]

Not long ago, the Colgan Institute, based near San Diego, analyzed 200 of the most commonly eaten foods for boron content and found that the daily intake of this trace mineral is just 1.9 milligrams—far below the minimum daily requirement of three milligrams.[16]

However, inasmuch as most people don't vary their diet beyond thirty different foods daily, they often miss many, if not most, of the foods richest in boron. Therefore, their daily intake of boron is estimated at a mere 0.35 to 0.42 of a milligram.

Why Boron Is Essential

Only within the last two decades has the importance of boron been realized. Drs. Curtiss Hunt and Forrest Nielsen, of the U.S. Department of Agriculture's Human Nutrition Research

Center in Grand Forks, North Dakota, demonstrated that boron is essential to good health.[17]

Boron provides hydroxyl groups vital to the synthesizing of certain steroid hormones, particularly those necessary for the metabolism of calcium, magnesium, manganese, and phosphorus in the bone and for muscle growth. Much fanfare has accompanied the use of boron—along with calcium, magnesium, manganese, silica, and vitamin D—to prevent osteoporosis or to cope with it.[18]

So far as preventing or coping with osteoporosis, biochemists generally agree that boron may slow down bone loss in postmenopausal women. Boron's role is twofold: it helps the body retain dietary calcium and it can increase the levels of natural estrogen.

Attention: Post-Menopausal Women

A study by Drs. Hunt and Nielsen followed twelve postmenopausal women on a very low intake of boron (0.25 milligrams daily) for seventeen weeks. They were found to have little active estrogen in their blood.

Then they were fed three milligrams of boron daily—the amount estimated to be adequate in a well-balanced diet—for seven weeks.

What happened was surprising and dramatic. Blood levels of estradiol-17B, the most active form of estrogen, doubled to "levels found in women on estrogen replacement therapy," according to Dr. Nielsen.

These levels were fifty percent higher than prestudy levels. Further, blood levels of testosterone, the precursor of estradiol, more than doubled. This is especially significant because these hormones are associated with strong, hard bones and teeth.[19]

A Substitute for Estrogen Replacement?

It is conceivable that boron supplementation may eventually become a natural alternative to synthetic estrogen replacement—or at least a supplement to it—in helping women cope with the various symptoms of menopause: bone-thinning characteristic of osteoporosis, breast reduction, clitoris shrinking, hot flashes, vaginal tissue thinning or even atrophy, and the skin's loss of sensitivity to touch.

"These steroid hormones are thought to be very important for maintaining bone and calcium status," stated Dr. Hunt, adding that he "suspects that the body needs boron to synthesize estrogen, vitamin D, and other steroid hormones. And it may also protect these hormones against rapid breakdown."[20]

Again referring to their study, the USDA scientists, said that, within eight days after the three-mg daily boron supplement was taken, the volunteers lost forty percent less calcium, thirty-three percent less magnesium, and slightly less phosphorus in their urine. Additionally, their calcium and magnesium losses were lower than those measured in the prestudy, when the women were on their usual diets.

"These elements are important in maintaining the integrity of bone," said Dr. Nielsen. "Boron had a remarkable effect on indicators that the body is conserving calcium and preventing bone demineralization. But we were really became excited when we saw its effect on steroid hormones."[21]

An Amazing Trace Mineral

Boron seems to help bone absorption when there is insufficient vitamin D intake through food and supplements and through exposure to sunlight. Nielsen and Hunt fed chickens a diet deficient in vitamin D, which should have stunted bone growth. However, boron supplementation renewed bone growth, and, once again, the chickens grew normally.

Nielsen and Hunt did a four-month follow-up study, which demonstrated that varying intakes of boron control the ability to retain calcium in bones and teeth, prompting Nielsen to announce the following:

"If more of the active form of calcium is retained in the blood, less is lost from the bone, which would be beneficial in preventing osteoporosis. I'm very encouraged about this calcium-conserving effect."[22]

Boron also seems to be effective in preventing arthritis and possibly in alleviating it. Robert M. Giller, M.D., reported that there seems to be a higher incidence of arthritis in areas where boron is deficient in the soil. He found two milligrams of boron daily helpful in treating arthritis patients. Boron and zinc seemed to reduce swelling in joints of his rheumatoid arthritis patients.[23]

Rave Reviews for Boron

A double-blind, eight-week study of twenty osteoarthritis patients conducted in the United Kingdom by Richard L. Travers, M.D. and associates, revealed that of ten patients on six milligrams of boron daily, five showed improvement, compared with only one of ten in the placebo group.[24]

Another bonus from the study was the finding that boron also influences how well the body conserves the key trace element copper. Copper helps in the producing of red blood cells and makes a major contribution to the function of the heart by keeping arteries healthy and protected against lesions, which often lead to accumulation of cholesterol and, eventually, blocked arteries.

One of the little-known aspects of boron is its effect on our ability to think efficiently, as highlighted by the studies of the USDA's James Penland, Ph.D., a research psychologist. Dr. Penland found that individuals deficient in boron show certain brain wave patterns, indicating that they are less alert. Their responses to stimuli are also slower, as is their motor coordination.[25]

A Powerful Brain Booster

What is the significance of this? Such brain waves are usually associated with people in their fifties and sixties, typical of normal aging. They are also common to people who are malnourished or exposed to toxins in the environment or food, such as lead.

"When you reduce dietary boron, you're almost certainly going to get a drop in alpha-wave activity and an increase in theta-wave activity from what I've seen on electroencephalograms (EEG)," stated Penland. "That's the same type of change you see when people become drowsy or less alert."

Dr. Penland conducted a revealing two-month study of fifteen individuals related to thinking and remembering. When this group ate chicken, mashed potatoes, rice, bread, and drank skim milk and had little fruit or vegetables, their brains showed a low boron content, and their ability to think and remember efficiently declined. Usually alert, they were now drowsy. When they were given a three-milligram boron supplement, their alertness, thinking, memory, perception, and attention span improved dramatically.[26]

Boron-containing seeds such as that of the chia plant bring us more benefits than just nourishment, the subject of the next chapter.

Seed Foods:
The Buffer Against Cancer

O NE OF THE WORLD'S FOREMOST AUTHORITIES ON SEEDS AND one of the most enthusiastic advocates of seed eating is Walter Troll, Ph.D., professor of environmental medicine at New York University. And he has good reason.

Back in 1969 he made his life's most momentous discovery: that an ingredient in seeds and nuts called protease inhibitors (PIs) actually can block the development of cancers by interfering with oncogenes. These are genes that potentially can change normal cells to cancerous cells and proteases that promote cancer.

"That day in 1969 is one I'll never forget," he told me. Why? Because his discovery offers a nontoxic way of coping with various kinds of cancers.[1]

Dr. Troll added protease inhibitors to a sure-fire cancer-causing solution that he painted on the skin of mice. No cancer developed, and Dr. Troll experienced the high of an incredible medical breakthrough.

The Wonder of PIs

Lab experiments revealed that PIs prevent the growth of human breast cancer and colon cancer cells. Protease inhibitors from seeds and beans fed to lab animals put the biochemical brakes on breast, colon, and skin cancers. Protease inhibitors injected into mice protect them from doses of normally lethal radiation.

But can protease inhibitors eaten in seeds, nuts, and legumes survive the acid hazards of a trip down the alimentary canal? "Absolutely," Dr. Troll told me. "I have traced them by radioactivity in animals, and they came out intact."

The powerful digestive juices in the stomach etch away the seed's outer coat, but, without question, the protease inhibitors are not destroyed or changed in the intestinal tract.

Although protease inhibitors are a blessing to mankind—womankind, too—they were included in seeds for another purpose: to make them an indestructible and indigestible curse to birds that eat them, Dr. Troll told me. Therefore, seeds are excreted whole by birds, so they can fall to earth and bring about new plants.

The ABCs

How do protease inhibitors block cancer? To get that answer, we must first know what proteases are and do. Proteases are enzymes that split protein into various amino acids.

There are scores of different oncogenes that live in normal cells. Usually they cause no harm, Dr. Troll said. However, when something causes them to mutate, turning them into cancer genes, they multiply almost uncontrollably and develop into a tumor.

Now oncogenes take part in the cells' initiation to cancer and to their progression into a tumor. One theory holds that free radicals can trigger oncogenes into life-threatening change. Free radicals, molecules with a missing electron, run amuck, capturing an electron from an adjoining molecule and turning that into a rapacious free radical that repeats the process in a destructive chain reaction. In damaging cell DNA, they may pull the trigger on resident oncogenes, changing them from peaceful guests into killers.

Little-Known Soldiers

Antioxidants quench free radicals and stop the wholesale injury or even total destruction of cells. Although the body synthesizes some antioxidants, many come in foods and supplements, indicated Dr. Troll.

Protease inhibitors are little known antioxidants that serve as palace guards who prevent free radicals from sabotaging our health. There's more. They also serve as internal surgeons who repair DNA damage and cut off the food supply to cancers, actually destroying them.

It is almost impossible for us to avoid the toxins in our environment. They assail us in the air we breathe, in the food we eat, and in the water we drink, creating free radicals that try to do us in. Even if the oncogenes are triggered, the protease inhibitors do some of their best work in keeping malignant cells from multiplying and spreading, stated Dr. Troll.

Revealing Research

Through an experiment with Seymour Garte, an associate researcher at New York University, Dr. Troll knows that oncogenes can definitely spark the start of cancer.

Garte and Troll took a certain type of oncogene—the ras gene—from the DNA of a human bladder cancer and planted it inside normal cells. Immediately, it started to multiply into cancerous cells. When the researchers inserted protease inhibitors, the cancerous changes stopped.[2]

Protease inhibitors are effective in the early stages of cancer, but do they work in later stages?

"Usually, yes," Dr. Troll told me. "They definitely slow down cancer growth even in later stages, all the way up to the time that the cancer spreads from its first site, the time of metastasizing. That's why I advocate eating foods rich in protease inhibitors for prevention."

The Kennedy Coup

Ann Kennedy, Ph.D., of the department of Radiation Oncology at the University of Pennsylvania, who has conducted a great deal of original work in protease inhibitors (some with Dr. Troll) made an awesome discovery while at the Harvard School of Public Health.

Many authorities on protease inhibitors have maintained that once a cell's genetic code has been changed by a cancer-causative, it cannot be reversed. However, in a test tube, Dr. Kennedy added protease inhibitors to tissue that had its genetic code altered and reversed the cancer-causing damage, bringing the DNA back to normal.[3]

Further, when Dr. Kennedy and associates added protease inhibitors—these from soybeans—to the diets of hamsters, they blocked mouth cancer. Added to the diet of mice, PIs stopped colorectal cancer. Dr. Kennedy is convinced that protease inhibitors can fight every type of cancer except that of the stomach.[4]

More Convincing Studies

There's still more evidence that seeds can help save you and me from cancer.

Pelayo Correa, Ph.D., of the Department of Pathology at Louisiana State University Medical Center in New Orleans, surveyed foods typically eaten in forty-one countries relative to cancer incidence. He found a heavy intake of seed foods in countries with the lowest rates of breast, colon and prostate cancer.[5]

It is a fact that protease inhibitors contain a certain amount of antioxidants. However, Dr. Correa notes that protease inhibitors are more potent cancer preventives than the usual antioxidants.

"The latter [protease inhibitors] may have an important advantage over the antioxidants in that test tube (in vitro) studies suggest that the protective effect of protease inhibitors lasts much longer," he writes. "Antioxidants, as a rule, cease to protect the subject or the cell when they are no longer present in abundant amounts."[6]

Dr. Pelayo writes that "on the cancer initiation and promotion side, emphasis has been placed mostly on macro-nutrient consumption (especially fat), carcinogens in food or produced by food processing, and contamination of food with carcinogens, either natural or synthetic (pesticides and the like). On the cancer inhibition side, most emphasis has been on fiber, antioxidant micronutrients, stimulators of immune defenses, and nonnutrient components of food. Protease inhibitors should be classified in the last category."[7]

A Difference of Opinion

Some researchers indicate that although protease inhibitors may block cancer in most body areas, they may be harmful to the pancreas. Dr. Ann Kennedy counters that argument:

"There are normal human populations with high levels of protease inhibitors in the diet which show no increased risk of pancreatic cancer: the Japanese and Seventh Day Adventists;

in fact, the Seventh Day Adventists have a decreased risk of developing pancreatic cancer, and we have observed no undesirable side effects.

"Thus, it is highly likely that protease inhibitor supplementation to the diet will prevent the development of cancer without adverse side effects in human populations."[8]

Dr. Troll adds that animal experiments give even more validity to Dr. Kennedy's findings. Monkeys, which have some physical similarities to human beings, don't develop pancreatic cancer when on protease inhibitors. Neither do mice or pigs. He mentions that some authorities find that seed foods may even block some of the negative effects of high-fat diets, believed to initiate hormone-regulated cancers.[9]

Over and above their protection against cancers, protease inhibitors seem also to guard against heart disease, states Dr. Troll. Populations that eat liberal amounts of foods containing protease inhibitors also have less cardiovascular disease. Why? Because PIs guard them against abnormal blood clotting.[10]

PIs and Viruses

There is still more protective virtuosity in protease inhibitors, in their help controlling harmful viruses that can cause illness and even shorten our lives, according to Dr. Troll. On the other hand, proteases, which are useful in regulating key metabolic functions, also activate certain viruses that attach to our cells, come to life, and take over the cell's genetic machinery, multiplying themselves.

Protease inhibitors thwart the protease enzymes from triggering the viruses, assuring that they're dead before they're alive, so they can be flushed out of the intestinal tract.

A Staged War that Never Happened

Researchers at Johns Hopkins University School of Medicine staged what might have been a micro-miniature war, Dr. Troll told me. They placed human rotaviruses that cause intestinal symptoms—diarrhea, gas, and stomach cramps—into test tubes along with a number of protease inhibitors (derived from soybeans) and human cells, letting them do their thing.

But the war never materialized, because the protease inhibitors wiped out the viruses' ability to get started. The viruses could not become activated to invade the human cells and take over.

Then the researchers conducted two experiments with mice. First, they supplied the animals with protease inhibitors and subsequently injected a virus into them. The protease inhibitors prevented the virus from taking hold. When they injected the virus first, the protease inhibitor wouldn't work. It took high dosages of protease inhibitors given a number of times to control the virus under these conditions. The message here is loud and clear: always keep the body supplied with a high level of protease inhibitors, Dr. Troll advised.

Superior to Drugs?

Many researchers theorize that protease inhibitors are more effective than present-day antiviral drugs, all of which come with side effects. Inasmuch as the drugs are all targeted to the genetic material in the cells, there is fear that they may throw a wrench into our genetic machinery, damaging it and, over a period of time, even contributing to cancer.

Dr. Troll told me that "the Western diet, consisting of much meat and a relatively low proportion of vegetables, appears responsible for a higher rate of breast, colon, and prostate cancer.

"In contrast, diets rich in rice, maize, and beans lower the incidence of human cancers, inasmuch as all seeds contain high concentrations of PIs."

Seeds: The Essence of Life

Dr. Troll informed me that, in addition to the protease inhibitors in chia, "there are many nutritional goodies enclosed in those little seeds."

A favorite Bible passage for seed researchers is "And God said, behold, I have given you every herb bearing seed which is upon the face of the earth, and every tree, in which is the fruit of the tree yielding seed; to you it shall be meat." (Gen. I.29)

The seed is the essence of life itself, the object in which wonders work. All the concentrated supernutrients necessary to promote life are stored there, waiting for soil, sunlight, and rain. The blueprint for the plant is in the seed as well as the kinds and amounts of concentrated food necessary for several days to form a root, stem, and leaves.

Amazing Stories about Seeds

Seeds can wait patiently to give birth—not just for a few years, but often for lifetimes. One of the most sensational stories of all time about seeds made headlines in many newspapers some years ago.

Seeds found by a Japanese archaeologist in a 4,000-year-old tomb sprouted when exposed to sunlight. They had been dormant there in a soil with heavy clay.[11] This is not an isolated incident.

During World War II an ancient Egyptian tomb in the Nile Valley near Dashur was bombed, and giant wheat seeds were found with the deceased. A young U.S. airman stationed in

Portugal was given thirty-six kernels of grain in 1949. He sent them back to his father, a wheat-growing farmer in north central Montana.

Planted and watered, the seeds sprouted, producing kamut, Egyptian wheat. Within six years, these nomad seeds multiplied into 1,500 bushels of a new kind of grain, ever growing in popularity for breakfast cereals.[12]

First Priority

Many decades ago an article in *Science* magazine revealed that seeds usually have a higher concentration of key nutrients than the plants grown from them. Scientists reason that seeds in fruits and vegetables have first priority in receiving delivery of essential nutrients, because they assure that the plant or tree will reproduce itself.[13]

An article by R.C. Collison in the *Journal of Industrial and Engineering Chemistry* reveals that the proportion of organic minerals to inorganic minerals is much higher in seeds than in the stem or leafy parts. Even when there are few organic minerals available in soil, a greater amount will be delivered to the seed.[14]

Still another experiment, this by researcher Thomas H. Mather more than a century ago (reported in *Scientific Agriculture*), showed that seeds actually reject chemical fertilizer. Only stalks and leaves accepted it.[15]

Some years ago, the late J.I. Rodale, founder of *Prevention* magazine and *Organic Farming,* wrote a letter of inquiry on this subject to Professor William A. Albrecht, chairman of the Department of Soils at the University of Missouri and one of the foremost researchers in organic growing.

Here is the essence of Dr. Albrecht's reply:[16]

The chemical composition of seeds does not fluctuate as widely as the chemical composition of vegetation. The seed is the means of survival of the species. This survival will not be possible unless a minimum of food materials is contained in the seed.

It is well established that when the fertility of the soil drops to a low level, less seed is produced. Seemingly, the amount of seed is the variable, while the quality of the seed is more nearly constant. The fertility of the soil as a growth-providing substance seems to determine the seed production, rather than the air, water, and sunshine that contribute the starches and the energy materials.

The fact that seeds appear to reject the synthetic fertilizers so widely used today and accept organic soil nutrients is an excellent reason for including more seeds in our diet, rather than concentrating on the stalks and leaves of the plant, which do accept synthetic fertilizers.

Luther Burbank's Opinion of Seeds

In an old book, *Partner of Nature,* Luther Burbank, the great plant wizard, made a significant statement about the infinite value of seeds, in contrast with the products that encase them:

"Fruits ripen, not to make food for us, but to encase the seeds inside—pips or pits or kernels. But we pay no attention to Nature's purpose and revel in the delicate flavors and delicious flesh of apples, pears, peaches, tomatoes, melons and all and throw aside carelessly the seeds that the plant went to so much trouble to build and in which it stored the life-giving germ and a reserve of starch to help it start in life again as a baby plant."

Amen!

CHAPTER 8

Domesticating the Wild Chia

T HOMAS JEFFERSON SAID IT, AND IT INSPIRED BOB ANDERSEN:

"No service can be rendered to a country that is more valuable than to introduce a new plant to the culture."

Bob Andersen's part (and Thomas Jefferson's indirectly), in helping to introduce kamut, Egyptian wheat, to the United States, excited him about the possibility of domesticating chia. (Bob worked with three members of the Quinn family to popularize kamut.)

"Twenty years ago, Hal Neiman was bringing chia seed in from Central America," says Andersen. "And I owned HealthBest and Organic Foods and Gardens, a company I bought from Hal.

"The latter company sold chia seeds to the natural food trade, distributors to health food stores and directly to the stores. HealthBest also sold to the natural foods trade.[1]

"So my company bought this chia seed from Hal and resold it. There weren't many people in the United States in that business then. Chia seed had been around for ages, and a lot of people knew about it, but there was so little of it. If you searched the world over, you might get 10,000 or 20,000 pounds in a year. And the following year, you might get nothing.

The Inside Story

"So then the Chia Pet people started their well-advertised and publicized sales campaign. Hal, the only chia seed importer at the time, sold them chia seeds he had bought from the Indians in Central America. The Chia Pet became increasingly popular and demanded a greater amount of seeds, which induced us to think in terms of developing even more product.

"Eventually, almost twenty years ago, Hal and I got together, because we had the connections in Central America. I wanted to do something with chia greater than had ever been done before—to develop a large and steady supply of it and introduce it to the American public.

"Hal and I had been friends for years. Because of my experience in helping to popularize kamut, I felt we knew how to introduce chia. So then came the struggle of learning how to mass grow and sell it.

"It's a funny story in some respects. We visited countries where it is grown and attempted to capture the market."

A Glaring Error

"In Central America, we talked to all the people who bought chia seed from the Indians there and then sold it. Here's what we accomplished the first year. By our great demand, we drove the price of chia seed up by two dollars a pound. There were little cells of people who sold it. When we told everybody in Guatemala City that we wanted to buy all the chia seed they had, the word really got around.

"One producer or dealer told the other, and we drove the price of chia seed so high that it cost us a fortune. We couldn't refuse to buy it. We had commitments. Then we had to figure out how we could swing the deals without driving our resale price through the roof."

The Awakening

"This devastating experience made us realize that we had to grow it ourselves. We met a man in Central America who volunteered to plant the chia seed in the wonderfully rich soil of a volcanic area. In the first year, disaster struck.

"Ants came and carried all the chia seed away. Ants like chia—they have very good taste—so we had no crop. We didn't fare much better the next year. Once the seeds were planted, the birds came and carried them away.

"To solve the ant problem, we moved to a higher altitude and then hired people to shoo away the birds. That was more economical and effective than installing machinery or setting up scarecrows throughout the vast acreage.

"An even bigger problem was how we could domesticate a plant that had grown wild. Over and above coping with the ant and bird problems, we had to learn characteristics of the chia plants.

"We found that the plants have to dry up totally before the seeds can be harvested. Then we beat the seeds out of the pods, which are somewhat like the rounds of sunflowers. Some chia plants we grow in the wild. We found low-cost ways of harvesting these seeds. Acreage that we domesticated kept costs from skyrocketing out of sight.

"Chia is so difficult to domesticate that until this day, we still have problems. So, as insurance for a regular and ample supply, we formed and control a network of independent farms. Native people—small families—grow corn way up in the hills on maybe less than a hectare of land. They grow chia seed between rows of corn.

"These small farms have developed chia as an alternative crop. The children, wives, and land owners gather the chia. The local government was very pleased about this, because it encouraged people to grow crops that would help them economically. Chia seeds could bring them two or three times what they made on corn."

Doing Business in Another Land

"When you travel on the backroads, you see little parcels of land," Anderson continued. "The story we heard about them follows. Say that Don Jose owned 100,000 acres and used it to ranch cattle. When he died, each of his ten children were willed one-tenth of the property. And then each one had ten children, and they each got one-tenth of it. So now there are little plots of land where the numerous great grandchildren of Don Jose have only a small fraction of the original acreage. This system of inheritance has changed the economics of the area.

"We feel good that we had the opportunity to help the small farmers, those who literally grow a crop in their back-yard and carry it down to the marketplace and sell it.

"The countryside is picturesque. You see these beautifully colored busses coming out of the mountains—gorgeous reds, blues, and oranges and whites—all decorated. Everyone of them has a name and is packed with passengers and their possessions. There are people hanging on the outside and sitting on the top. Native pedestrians on the roadside carry baskets of fruits, nuts, and chia seed to sell in the marketplace."

Our Knowledge Grows

"We've developed a network of representatives who buy directly from these small growers," Anderson told me. "We now have enough people to gather the chia, and we're even getting a lot of product from the wild crop. Then we also joined with a group of more sophisticated farmers in South

America. They were receiving advice from the University of California at Davis and the University of Arizona.

"What happened on the experimental plots was a learning experience. At the very beginning, we needed help and advice from the universities. This involved guiding the natives in converting a wild crop to a domesticated crop without changing the character of the seed and learning how and where to grow it and under what conditions so that we could row-crop it. It must be planted every year, because animals love the seed and eat whatever remains on the ground.

"In the wild, the chia plant just grows from its own seeds that drop to the ground. We are now experimenting, planting crops at various altitudes, in various types of soil, and in many different countries, trying to find where it grows best. It does like a tropical climate."

Certain Types Are Hard to Harvest

"The type of seeds that we mainly grow, the *Salvia hispanica,* thrives in higher altitudes and loves a climate such as you'll find in Central America. We're not growing the *Columbaraie,* the golden chia, due to results from an experiment we conducted on a couple of acres just outside Murrieta on Gentry's Experimental Farm in southern California. Gentry's son-in-law, the gentleman who runs it now, Peter McKown—a real advocate of chia—and about twenty of us met to harvest that acre. We worked for three hours and harvested a mere thirty pounds.

Harvesting costs would be so high that the retail sale price of chia seed would be prohibitive for most consumers. This is why it is difficult to grow and harvest chia seed in the U.S.

"We found that people who had a good agricultural background and the willingness and time to study the plant did the best growing for us. Now, for the first time, we have an adequate supply of chia seed. We have only sold to people who were purchasers from the past, including the Chia Pet group and others of our regular distributors.

"We are excited about an opportunity for everyone to learn about chia as a food, because most people only know about chia as a novelty through the Chia Pet."

Chia Seed: Now Market-Ready

"It is reassuring to us that, after all these years of trial and error in growing chia seed, we're in a position to assure companies interested in the benefits and marketability of it that we will have the product—the important thing that we couldn't do before.

"We are now where we want to be. The challenge of knowing how to grow it, where to grow it, and how to harvest it successfully without ruining the seed is, fortunately, behind us. Now we have to open the eyes of consumers to the value they can find in this little seed—the wonderful energy, endurance, and enhanced nutrition.

"We are still looking for alternative growing places for chia throughout Central and South America. Eventually we may grow the seed on all continents in the world. Growers in Vietnam and China are eager for more information. Recently a company from China wrote us of its interest in experimenting with chia. Our objective, of course, is to increase the world supply to get the price down to where it is affordable to as many people as possible."

Striking Oil in Chia Seeds

"Then we will start processing the oil—a big, big product. It is a healthful oil for all kitchen purposes—cooking, baking, or tossing with salads. Its ratio of linolenic to linoleic acid is more favorable than oil from any other seed or grain. Further, it oxidizes more slowly than any other oil.

"Then there are also uses for chia seed oil beyond food and nutrition. Chia seed oil is a wonderful product to apply to oil paintings. It preserves the paintings, and they remain clear and don't change colors.

"The Indians of Central and South America, and even up into this area, also used chia oil to preserve wood products. It saturates the wood and preserves it against the elements. One of the potential uses for this is as a polish for furniture.

"We think that the uses for chia seed oil are beyond immediate comprehension. We haven't even scratched the surface yet."

Not Just for Athletes

"Imagine the idea just thrown across the table to me today by a sports doctor. Chia seed is a hydrophilic colloid. It is a substance that absorbs a great amount of water and becomes a gelatinous mass in your stomach. If you're running and it slowly disperses that mass into your system, you're going to have longer-lasting energy than the person who doesn't have that advantage.

"This is at least a partial answer to the energy and endurance imparted by chia. And low energy is a problem for most people. Fatigue is the major problem that patients present to their doctors.

"Dehydration is a big problem for athletes as well as laborers in torrid equatorial zones. So chia seed can help to cope with this problem and many others."

A Great Adventure

"Our adventure in Central and South America has been the fact that a lot of emerging nations there and elsewhere are looking for an alternative crop—something that opens a new market. We just have to wake up the American spirit and get it out there.

"Imagine, here's a product with all those remarkable ingredients. It's a rare seed, and if companies were to use it in their products and promote it, they would have a ground-floor opportunity. In a competitive world we like to be the first company or group of companies to have access to such a product.

"It is, of course, feasible to grow chia seed in the southwestern United States. After all, that's where it grows wild. We are experimenting with it. However, we have not, as yet, found a way to harvest it economically. The kind that grows best in these desert areas is the *Columbariae*, whose seeds are very difficult to gather and, therefore, prohibitively costly to harvest.

"The *Columbariae* doesn't come in a pod. There are seeds imbedded in many holes with flesh-piercing spikes all around them, so harvesting is tedious and painful. And the more harvestable *Hispanica* won't grow well in the southwestern desert.

"Well, these words cover the high spots of our adventure growing chia. Soon people all over the world will be eating it and benefitting from it. I hope Thomas Jefferson would have been pleased with us."

CHAPTER 9

Real Foods for Real People

IN A LAND SO RICH IN HEALTH-GIVING CHIA—AS WELL AS OTHER nutrition-rich plants—it is disturbing that the health of Native Americans in the southwestern desert is diminished by obesity, fatigue, frequent illnesses and infections, gum diseases, cavities and pyorrhea, and, particularly, type II diabetes.

As *New York Times* columnist Jane Brody pointed out, this is simply because they have deserted healthful native foods for modern, nutrition-poor, processed foods. There's a health lesson to be learned by all of us here.

The sharp decline in Indian heath began in the early 1940s with World War II. The Pimas and other tribes left their reservations, home gardens, and native foods to add to their meager U.S. government subsidies by working in cotton fields or in war-related factories or by joining the armed forces.

Immediately they were exposed to nutrient-poor, processed foods high in calories and refined carbohydrates (sugar and starch) and loaded with fats.

Devastating Results

Between the war and 1970, the weight of the average Pima shot up by ten pounds, often to a level of obesity. Obesity is a high-risk factor for adult-onset diabetes (type II).

An outcry of Native Americans and their neighbors brought health researchers from Washington to help the O'Odhams (also known as the Papagos and Pimas) and all tribes of the area.

However, these investigators, deeply indoctrinated with orthodox beliefs, failed to understand the causes: the starch- and sugar-rich, nutrient-poor processed food brought onto the reservations by the U.S. government and into stores near the reservations and, in addition, the inactive life of the O'Odhams.

Misunderstood Problems

A few paragraphs by Gary Nabhan from a quarterly newsletter issued by Native Seeds/SEARCH, of Tucson, Arizona, fully explains this failure:

"Despite a twenty-year, multimillion-dollar effort by the National Institutes of Health and the Indian Health Service to study the causes and cures of this disease, little effort has been given to understanding the relationship of the O'Odhams' traditional diet to diabetes.

"The NIH/IHS team apparently lost interest in traditional diet composition after a 1971 study suggested that the average O'Odham today consumes about the same number of calories, and the same amounts of carbohydrates and fat as the average U.S. citizen. But that dietary study, like others, failed to analyze the actual traditional foodstuffs that comprised the O'Odham diet historically.

"It simply substituted known nutritional values of conventional analogs for the native foods. For example, any kind of dry bean, whether tepary, pinto or lima, was considered the same as the dry beans listed in standard USDA food composition tables."[1]

A Challenge to Erroneous Assumptions

Researcher David Jenkins challenged this assumption, often offered by dieticians advising diabetics. It confirmed that the carbohydrate exchange lists offered by the American Diabetic Association and other groups did not reflect the true physiological effects of foods in reducing blood sugar levels after eating.

"Jenkins developed a glycemic index, a measure of effects of different foods on blood glucose," writes Nabhan. "The lower the score on the index, the greater the benefits to diabetics and those suffering from hypoglycemia (low blood sugar). He found that the foods having the least negative effects in the diabetic diets were those commonly eaten by nondominant cultures—ethnic minorities in the west and many land-based communities in the Third World.

"Jenkins and collaborators were tempted to conclude that diabetes is a disease of adopting the values and diets of dominant affluent cultures, which are dysfunctional for the metabolisms of many ethnic populations throughout the world," concludes Nabhan.[2]

Gary Nabhan's Mighty Contribution

When governmental agencies failed to solve Native Americans' serious health problems and quietly backed away, Gary Nabhan, a desert ecologist-conservationist with a heart for the land, its seeds, and the people, saw a simple solution.[3]

Native Americans suffered mass sickness because they had stopped growing and eating nourishing desert foods to which they had been accustomed for thousands of years.[4]

Nabhan understood other reasons for the Native Americans' ill health and wretched state. Funding for Indian affairs was never ample. Entire families struggled desperately to subsist on less than $4,000 annually. Doctors were scarce and rarely closer than fifty miles away. And few patients could afford a car or bus transportation to and from a town or city.[5]

Nabhan had been active in recovering native food crop seeds that had been grown for thousands of years and were in danger of being lost forever. He began to realize that his work extended beyond recovering precious endangered seeds of desert plants and included helping Native Americans recover their health, well-being, morale, and dignity.

Success Through Cooperation

Nabhan directed his attention to epidemic illnesses of Native Americans. At the same time, Jean Brand, a nutritionist at the University of Sydney and other Australian scientists had discovered a similar problem in the deteriorating health of aborigines in the Land Down Under. The two agreed to work together.

Nabhan sent Brand six typical Pima foods of the past, which were fed to eight nondiabetic Caucasians. A control group of matched individuals ate typical processed Western meals—potatoes, white enriched bread, and processed cereals—a diet heavy in refined sugar and starches. The intake of calories was equal in both groups.

Findings hammered home the answer to why the Pimas suffered such a high level of diabetes. The first group, eating native foods, showed a controlled blood sugar response and a consistent level of blood glucose, key factors in preventing the start of adult-onset diabetes.

In sharp contrast, the typical Western foods brought on quick, high-blood-sugar responses. Then Brand's comparative analysis of both diets, equal in amounts of starches, brought out the real significance of the study. The Western diet had quick-release carbohydrates, while the Pima diets had slow-release carbohydrates high in amylose, a starch that breaks down slowly into simple sugars and contributes to greater energy and endurance.

The Willoughby Analysis

In a remarkable article, "Primal Prescription," John Willoughby summed up the principle of slow release carbohydrate power in terms of chia seeds, as demonstrated to him by Gary Nabhan:

"Nabhan placed a spoonful of the tiny black chia seeds in a glass of water. When he returned to his house later, the glass appeared to contain not seeds and water, but an almost solid gelatin. This gelatin-forming activity is due to the soluble fiber in chia seed," Nabhan explained.[6]

Brand and other researchers believe that this same gel-forming phenomenon takes place in the stomach when foods containing these mucilages are eaten. The gel formed in the stomach then creates a physical barrier between carbohydrates and the digestive enzymes that break them down, slowing the conversion of carbohydrates into sugar.

This phenomenon explains the ability of chia to give strength and endurance to athletes who eat it regularly and as a part of the complex of foods acting as a preventive against diabetes.

Verified Findings

Willoughby cites a confirming study by Dr. Boyd Swinburn at the Indian Hospital in Phoenix. Twenty-two healthy nondiabetics were fed a reconstructed diet of the Pimas of 1870 for fifteen days, then switched back to a modern, high-fat, refined-carbohydrate diet of equal calories.

Volunteers showed no blood-sugar stresses when eating native foods. However, the volunteers on the modern Western diet experienced quicker and greater blood sugar increases and a lesser ability of insulin to reduce that sugar. Swinburn concluded from this that a return to the native diet would protect the Pimas, with their genetic predisposition to diabetes, from the actual disease.

There's more about this problem and its solutions in the following chapter.

The Price Studies

The research of Gary Nabhan, although on a small scale, reminds me of the monumental, long-term studies done by the late Weston A. Price, D.D.S, reported in his classic book, *Nutrition and Physical Degeneration,* now distributed exclusively by the Price-Pottenger Foundation in La Mesa, California.

During the 1930s Dr. Price toured the world to visit people living in pockets protected from the full impact of processed foods: inhabitants of the Loeschental Valley of Switzerland, natives of the Outer Hebrides, Eskimos of Alaska, Melanesians and Polynesians of the South Pacific, tribes in central and eastern Africa, aborigines of Australia, the Maori of New Zealand, and ancient civilizations of Peru and the Amazon basin.

Price examined, studied, and photographed native groups who had never eaten processed and debilitated Western foods such as refined sugar and flour and those who had eaten them for more than a generation.

Frightening Results from Fractionated Foods

In second-generation individuals on Western foods, he found narrowing faces and dental arches, causing crowded teeth and tooth decay; smaller nostrils, making breathing more difficult;

and narrowed pelvic girdles, which made giving birth more stressful and painful.

Those who stayed with native whole foods were just the opposite—picture-book examples of excellent appearance, with ample facial and dental arches and pelvic girdles.

Asked if it usually took several generations for deterioration to happen, Dr. Price said "not always."

Disturbances developed in these groups starting in the first generation after the adoption of the modern diet and rapidly increased in severity, displaying the characteristic degenerative processes of our modern American and European cultures.

Sources of These Problems

Dr. Price indicated that certain physical defects were directly related to inadequate nutrition of the mother during the formative period of the fetus. However, his research reveals that the problem goes back still further.

In many groups, Dr. Price found that traditionally girls were not allowed to be married until after a period of special feeding. In some tribes, six months of special nutrition was required before marriage.

Dr. Price's discoveries were saluted by a prominent anthropologist, Dr. Earnest Hooton of Harvard University, in the book's foreword:

"Dr. Price has accomplished one of those epochal pieces of research which make every investigator desirous of kicking himself because he never thought of doing the same thing.... Dr. Price found out why primitive people have good teeth and why their teeth go bad when they become 'civilized.' But he has not stopped there. He has gone on to apply his knowledge acquired from primitive people to the problems of their less intelligent civilized brothers.

"For I think that we must admit that if primitive people know enough to eat the things which keep their teeth healthy, they are more intelligent in dietary matters than we are."

Although Dr. Weston Price is no longer with us, his immense contribution to good health and well-being still live in *Nutrition and Physical Degeneration* and in the Price-Pottenger Foundation in La Mesa, California.

This unique organization carries on his principles and those of the late Francis M. Pottenger, Jr., M.D. (The 525-page sixth edition of *Nutrition and Physical Degeneration* can be obtained for $19.95 and a $6.00 shipping and handling charge from the Price-Pottenger Foundation, P.O. Box 2614, La Mesa, CA 91943-2614; phone (619) 574-7763; fax (619) 574-1314).

CHAPTER 10

Back to the Past

Some statistics are unbelievable. Some are frightening. Some are even true. The ones you are about to see are unbelievable, frightening, *and* true. Prior to World War II, diabetes was no more common among the O'Odham tribes of Arizona than in the typical American community. Twenty-five years later, the prevalence of diabetes there is fifteen times that of the typical American community.[1]

What follows is important not only to Native Americans but to people the world over who have diabetes or who, sometimes even unknowingly, may be in danger of developing it.

Gary Nabhan relates that more than half of the O'Odham over thirty-five years old have adult-onset diabetes—one of the highest diabetes rates in the world. Other Indian tribes are right behind them statistically.[2]

There are 250,000 diabetics among the Arizona Indians. "It's a nightmare," says Nabhan. Soon these diabetics in Arizona "will cost taxpayers a minimum of $320 million a year. If adopted at an early age, nutritional intervention such as selected native foods may reduce health costs and suffering now impacting Indians genetically susceptible to diabetes."[3]

Reversal of a Serious Disease

The story of Earl Ray, a Pima tribesman who lives in a small trailer on the Salt River reservation, not far from Phoenix, exemplifies what happens to Native Americans who eat highly processed foods rather than native whole foods, such as chia seeds and other desert products. It also illustrates what can happen to anybody anywhere addicted to junk foods.[4]

Earl Ray, as a five-foot six-inch adult, weighed between 145 and 150 pounds. Then he switched to eating largely fast foods—hamburgers, pizzas, packaged and processed food—and alcohol. He rapidly gained poundage until he weighed 239 and was diagnosed with severe diabetes.

Several years ago, Ray became acutely aware of his problem and made the hard decision to go back to Pima foods: chia, tepary beans, mesquite, cholla buds, prickly pears, Emory oak acorns, and chaparral tea. Today he weighs a slender 150 pounds, and his diabetes is under control. Explaining the slow release of energy from native desert foods, he tells those who comment on his physical transformation:

"It's kind of like taking a Contac cold tablet. It releases energy over an eight-hour period, in contrast to a candy bar, where you get burned out in an hour."

Remarkable Recovery

Ray also claims that natural desert foods reversed his hair loss brought on by diabetes, improved his teeth, got rid of his frequent stomachaches, and eased the discomfort of his arthritis.

Weston Price's finding that "modernized food" can contribute to diabetes is not unique to Earl Ray and residents of the southwestern desert.

The story of Somasundaram Addanki, a native of India and an associate professor of biochemistry and nutrition at Ohio State University, offers a similar message.

Addanki and his wife did not develop diabetes until they had left India and were regularly eating "a typical western diet."

In a United Press International article, Professor Addanki admitted to six years of diabetes and diabetic impotency prior to stopping eating refined sugar and products containing it, white flour products, and fatty foods.

When he went back to whole food—fresh fruits and vegetables with live enzymes as well as whole grains—he managed his diabetes and returned to good health.[5]

Diabetes Now Declining

Slowly the incidence of diabetes is declining in the southwest, thanks largely to Gary Nabhan and his associates at Native Seeds/SEARCH (NS/S). More and more gardeners and farmers grow Indian crops, writes NS/S staff member Kevin Dahl:

"Much of this interest is stimulated by the recognition that modern crop varieties require too much water to be economic in the Southwest. In the last twelve years, twenty percent of Arizona's cultivated land has been abandoned due to the high cost of pumping irrigation water."[6]

The primary mission of (NS/S) is to find, preserve, multiply, and disseminate seeds of native crops and to revive what remains of ancient ways and means of Southwestern horticulture.

"Integral to the preservation of seeds is the preservation of Native American cultures that have evolved with the crops themselves—each nurturing the other," writes Dahl.

"Specifically, the goals of NS/S are to preserve specific genetic types, support the conservation of lands where wild crop relatives are found, and promote the understanding and appreciation of traditional agricultural systems of Native

Americans in the Southwestern United States and northern Mexico."[7]

Native Seeds/SEARCH, a nonprofit, tax-exempt organization, is alive and growing, thanks to Meals for Millions, which initially helped Gary Nabhan establish a regional seed bank and conservancy garden. When Nabhan couldn't acquire enough seeds from native growers to fulfill requests, he decided to grow them.

Originally granted $25,000 by the Ruth Mott Fund, NS/S accepts contributions to carry on its work and has a membership above 2,500. The organization sells a catalogue that includes seeds for sale—1,200 varieties of heirloom seeds members have collected—and information on how to save seeds from each crop.[8]

In a sense, anyone who plants these seeds becomes a part of Native Seeds/SEARCH's mission. You can contact this organization at 2509 N. Campbell Avenue, #325, Tucson, Arizona 85719.

In recognition of his unique contribution to humankind, Gary Nabhan, a widely heralded ethnobiologist and natural historian, was recently awarded one of the MacArthur Foundation Fellowships—informally called "a genius fellowship." Its considerable financial stipend permits him total freedom to develop and pursue his own ideas.

Early Education to Combat Disease

One of Nabhan's projects, carried out through Native Seeds/SEARCH, is educating Pima children beginning in the first grade about the natural food treasures in their environment: chia, various types of Indian corn, mesquite seeds (often called "desert candy"), native squash, tepary beans, cholla buds, and Emory oak acorns.

The children are taught how to gather and prepare desert foods, so hundreds of years of tradition are being recaptured. And the health of the Pimas is already improving, as their unwanted weight vanishes along with symptoms of illness.

At least once a year, as part of its Diabetics Program, Native Seeds/SEARCH sponsors a native foods event for Pima students at various elementary schools.

Back to Native Foods

More than 200 students sit down to a Harvest Meal of squash soup, turkey, tepary beans, corn tortillas, spinach salad, prickly pear dressing, watermelon, acorns, and chia seeds, as well as a form of desert jello made from wild chia seed mixed with desert fruit and the bright purple prickly pear juice.[8]

On the day following the Harvest Meal, NS/S Education Director Martha Burgess and other staff members bring in of mesquite pods, tepary beans, native squash, colorful popcorn, acorns, and chia seeds, and the children are instructed by kitchen demonstration how to prepare the native foods.

They grind chia seeds to a powder with a stone mortar and pestle for various dishes or pop chia seeds into their mouths and "marvel at the explosion of the seeds and their jello-like texture." They are also invited to chew mesquite bean pods or grind them.

Gruesome Consequences of Junk Foods

"Once the children are hooked on the good tastes from these interesting new (to them) foods," says Martha Burgess, "our message of good energy and good health, like a cherished seed, can be planted with the hope of germination."[9]

As part of the lesson, one of the instructors usually asks the class, "Do you know what happens when you eat too much sugar?"

Inasmuch as most of the children have seen the results of complications from diabetes, neuropathies that can lead to impaired leg circulation, gangrene, and amputations, one eight-year-old boy immediately answered:

"They cut your legs off."

A Lesson for Everybody

The message to the children is to avoid refined sugar and fats and eat native foods high in soluble fiber—chia seeds, cholla buds and acorns—to avoid diabetes, neuropathies, and their gruesome consequences.

NS/S staff members have put together an exciting curriculum package to reinforce Harvest Meal and follow-up demonstrations: videos, slide/tape programs, and brochures packed with recipes for meals and snacks and nonsugared soft drink alternatives. Of course, seeds are part of the package, so children can practice planting, nurturing plant growth, harvesting, and tasting the finished products.

Prevention is the theme—prevention that will build strong bodies, electric energy, and endurance and, best of all, guard against diabetes and its painful, often devastating, consequences.

CHAPTER 11

Creativity with Chia

THE WRITINGS OF DR. WESTON PRICE AND THE SIGNIFICANT contributions of Gary Nabhan and Native Seeds/SEARCH deeply moved and motivated Linda Barrett and William Anderson to help to improve the quality of American fare.

They founded Menu 4 Life in Paso Robles, California. They wanted to return native quality and nutrition to modern foods, starting with school cafeteria fare.[1]

Dramatic results had been produced by many idealistic school nutritionists who had eliminated junk foods from cafeterias and had demonstrated with whole and natural foods that children could benefit in body, mind, and spirit.

A most impressive record had been attained some years before by Gena Larson, the nutritionist at Helix High School in La Mesa, California, in the greater San Diego area. (Gena was one of my columnists when I edited *Let's Live* magazine.) Wholesome cafeteria foods boosted grades and contributed to more competitive athletic teams and, in the process, resulted in far fewer broken bones and faster healing of those that did break.

Better Foods, Better Learning

Even more convincing to Linda and Bill was an in-depth, three-year study by Stephen Schoenthaler, Ph.D., Walter Doraz, and James Wakefield, Jr., of California State University, Stanislaus.[2]

They showed that an enhanced school diet contributed to higher grades for one million New York City public elementary and junior high school students, who were evaluated before and after school lunches were improved.

Dramatic rises in academic scores surprised school officials. Within four years after the school lunch program was upgraded, average test scores of 803 schools rose by fifteen percent.

At the study's launching (1979), New York City public schools ranked in the thirty-ninth percentile as rated by the standardized California Achievement Test scores used throughout the nation. This indicated that sixty-one percent of the nation's other school systems scored higher.

One year later, the New York City Board of Education reduced the sugar content of foods and prohibited the use of two artificial food colorings in school lunches. Later that year, achievement test scores rose sharply—this time to the forty-seventh percentile nationwide.[2]

Progressive Reforms

Deeply impressed with this gain, New York City public school officials outlawed foods with artificial coloring and flavoring. The result? Again, test scores moved upward—this time to the fifty-first percentile.

Trying to make a good thing even better, school officials banned foods containing two common preservatives: BHA and BHT. Once more, city school scores rose—now to the fifty-fourth percentile.

Next, junk foods were banned, with milk replacing carbonated soft drinks and candy. Over the span of the study, New York schools achieved more than a fifteen percentile academic gain. This resulted in a tremendous savings of school funding, because the schools required fewer special-education teachers to give individual instruction to children with reading problems.

The study by Schoenthaler and associates revealed typical mind/body saboteurs in the American diet: excessive sugar and artificial additives, including food colorings (many derived from coal tar, a carcinogenic substance), emulsifiers and preservatives.

Reform the Nation's School Menus

Bill Anderson, in collaboration with Linda Barrett and Rod Blackner, food services director of the Paso Robles School District, created a comprehensive school lunch program called Solutions, in response to a significant study by Tufts University. This study "confirms the link between nutrition and cognitive development in children," and shows that "even short term nutritional deficiencies influence children's behavior, ability to concentrate and perform complex tasks."[3]

The hunger of children during the early years often produces a lifetime of learning handicaps and impairments. An illusion that deserves shattering is the prevailing belief that such impediments affect only children of low-income families, who can't afford nutritious foods.

"Substandard nutritional intake of children in families on all economic and social levels is a silent enemy that undermines incentive to learn, learning, and remembering," says Bill Anderson.

Even before it is severe and results are readily detectable, deficient nutrition limits the ability of children to take in new information about the world around them.

Undernourished bodies conserve the limited food values available—first, to maintain critical organ functions; second, for growth; and third for social activity and cognitive development.

Undernourished bodies also impair children's ability to relate to one another, dull their inquisitiveness, extinguish their fire to learn, and reduce their attentiveness and, in time, their self-esteem. These losses are precursors to becoming school dropouts.

The Anderson-Barrett-Blackner Solutions is a systematic approach that goes beyond educating students about the value of good nutrition to educating parents, teachers, school administrators, and the community. It is an abrupt, ice-water awakening to the refreshing honesty that all segments of society are responsible for enhancing education.

How much more could be achieved by upgrading school menus with super-nourishing foods in addition to eliminating harmful foods and additives? Linda and Bill asked themselves.

Their company, Menu 4 Life, develops and produces chia seed recipes for a comprehensive school lunch program.

Bill and Linda have donated their unique garden bread recipes to Paso Robles schools, along with their time in production and consulting. In addition to working to produce breads for the school lunch program, Rod Blackner plans to market Linda and Bill's bread base wet ingredients—beans, oats, chia gel, vegetable or fruit, herbs, and spices—to other school districts.

In order to use the bread base, the schools need only add flour and yeast to produce a ready-to- bake dough for breads, bagels, pizzas, and rolls. This same base can also be used to produce a variety of flavored soups and pastas. For making fresh pastas, the schools would only need to add semolina flour.

In addition to using the base for bread doughs and pastas, Rod is using it for a great variety of soup starters. (Recipes are included on the packaging.) Rod is working with Menu 4 Life to produce additional chia products, including Bill and Linda's latest development, Chia Boost Formula, a nutritious snack product made into a gel pack, drink, and chewy fruit bar.

These prototype products have been tested extensively with groups of children and many student athletes with overwhelmingly positive results and are now on deck for production.

A two-year study of the program at one school site proved that the program is practical. Bill and Linda made classroom presentations and samplings of their breads and led tours through the kitchen when the dough was being prepared and the breads baked. They shared information about chia use by Native Americans. This led to a thirty-percent increase in consumption of the Garden Breads above schools in the rest of the district.

Bill Anderson and Linda Barrett encourage and challenge readers of this book to investigate their local schools' nutritional programs and question the content of their lunch program.

"If there is a question about the quality of the school lunch program and there is a need for the Solutions program, you are invited to contact me as to how to implement it in your school district," says Bill.

"Remember, if we are not all working and acting upon Solutions to this problem, we are, in fact, a part of the problem."

With the goal to upgrade the ability of students to learn and retain their knowledge and retain or build radiant good health and well-being, Menu 4 Life is open to consulting with

THE MAGIC OF CHIA

other school districts throughout the nation to develop similar programs. Linda and Bill can be reached at Menu 4 Life, P.O. Box 2693, Paso Robles, CA 93446, or by e-mail at menu4life@juno.com.

They can also supply additional information on chia seed, more recipes, available chia products, and an order for chia seed at a wholesale price. Chia seed is sold by the pound, and there are approximately 800,000 seeds in a pound.

An Idealistic Program

Any profits to Menus 4 Life will help to finance a culinary academy for health education and a work experience program for interested students.

Already underway, this academy has students planting gardens at various school sites for growing, nurturing, and harvesting foods and herbs. They are playing a key part in supplying foods served in the school lunch program and overcoming resistance to accepting and eating healthful foods.

The Staff of Life

Overhauling the full spectrum of American food was too mammoth a task for openers, so Linda and Bill started modestly with a single food: bread. Bread was originally made with whole grains rich in multinutrients from its bran and germ. But most bread is now made with refined white flour and is mainly starch, with a host of chemical additives.

Once the staff of life, over the years bread has become a broken crutch. Supposedly some synthetic vitamins and a few minerals are thrown in to compensate for the two dozen natural vitamins and organic minerals removed in flour processing.

One of the worst problems with nutritionally bankrupt foods is that the body senses it is being short-changed. Then, at the subconscious level, it drives us to eat more than we should, often causing us to gain unwanted weight. Our attention is often drawn to the word "enriched" on certain products. "Enriched" is an inaccurate word to characterize the addition of synthetic supplements to dead foods. "Deimpoverished" would be closer to the truth.

How does this relate to chia? In a big way! Here is a supernutritious food that represents a giant step back to the future—back to real food for real people and really good health.

Linda and Bill wanted a rebirth of bread to incorporate old, natural, health-giving ingredients.

"We start with unbleached wheat flour," Linda told me. "This is because many people who need nutritious bread most would reject a whole-grain bread. Then we combine that with yeast and chia seed and a wide range of other supernutritious foods.

"Garden Breads are made with half the flour contained in conventional breads. The other half is a combination of pureed, sprouted, cooked beans, oats, vegetables or fruit, chia gel, and a small amount of salt, yeast, and honey," explains Linda. "The garden breads need approximately half the yeast of most breads. We believe this is due to the abundant nutrients feeding the yeast.

"We now also have a perfected whole kamut (Egyptian wheat) loaf. It is made with plumped kamut berries and is a beautiful garden loaf, containing complete protein with abundant fiber, along with soluble fiber from soybean, oats, and chia gel.

"We begin our Garden Bread doughs with the bean, oat, chia gel, and vegetable or fruit mixture and add only enough flour to bring it all to dough consistency. Then we combine that and yeast with a wide range of super-nutritious foods."

Linda and Bill's combinations of ingredients are unique. No one had previously had the imagination to include them in bread. Familiar with the colorful history of chia seed and its ability to contribute to energy and endurance, they designed mouth-watering loaves that include chia as a major ingredient and as a topping used like caraway or poppy seed. Unlike most seed toppings, chia seed stays put and prevents drying out of the breads, by trapping its moisture with its hydrophilic fibers.

Meal in a Loaf

Garden Variety Breads carry the slogan "Meal in a Loaf." They come in eighteen different varieties, all accenting chia seed: Original Bean, Indian Chia, Frijole Jalapeno, "Guida" Sicilian, Rosemary Olive, Potato Chive, Chia Maize, Garbanzo Carrot, Oriental Garlic, Yam 'n' Yellow, Garden Loaf, Cajun Spice, Apple-Cinnamon-Raisin-Walnut, Banana Nut, Cocoa Bean, Pumpkin Lentil, Sweet Peach, and Lentil Sweet Potato.

Here are the ingredients of the breads. (Chia gel is water-soaked chia seed in a ratio of nine parts water to one part chia seed. This ratio mixture can be used in all of your baked goods recipes to replace oil.)

Original Bean: unbleached wheat flour, Great Northern white beans, cooked oats, chia gel, yeast, sea salt, and unprocessed honey.

Indian Chia: unbleached wheat flour, Great Northern white beans, cooked oats, beets, chia gel yeast, sea salt, and unprocessed honey.

Frijole Jalapeno: unbleached wheat flour, cooked pinto beans and oats, jalapeno peppers, chia gel, yeast, sea salt, and unprocessed honey. (This has an incredible south-of-the-border flavor and is one of my favorites.)

"Guida" Sicilian: unbleached wheat flour, cooked black beans and cooked oats, tomatoes, onions, chia gel, yeast, sea salt, molasses, herbs, and spices.

Rosemary Olive: unbleached wheat flour, Great Northern white beans, cooked oats, black olives, chia gel yeast, sea salt, and fresh rosemary.

Potato Chive: unbleached wheat flour, cooked Great Northern white beans and cooked oats, whole Idaho potatoes, green onion chives, chia gel, yeast, sea salt, and unprocessed honey.

Garbanzo Carrot: unbleached wheat flour, cooked garbanzo beans, oats, carrots, chia gel, yeast, sea salt, and unprocessed honey.

Oriental Garlic: unbleached wheat flour, cooked soy beans, oats, purple and green cabbage, chia gel, garlic, yeast, sea salt, liquid aminos, and unprocessed honey.

Yam 'n' Yellow: unbleached wheat flour, cooked yellow split peas, oats, baked whole yams, chia gel, yeast, sea salt, and unprocessed honey.

Garden Herb Loaf: unbleached wheat flour, cooked green split peas and oats, spinach, chia gel, yeast, sea salt, and unprocessed honey. (One or more of kale, collard greens, bok choy, or mustard can be substituted for spinach.)

Cajun Spice: unbleached wheat flour, cooked black-eyed peas, oats, potatoes, hominy, tomatoes, chia gel, yeast, sea salt, unprocessed honey, herbs, and spices.

Apple, Cinnamon, Raisin, Walnut: unbleached wheat flour, cooked Great Northern white beans and oats, whole apples, chia gel, raisins, walnuts, yeast, sea salt, unprocessed honey, cinnamon, and Tahitian vanilla.

Banana Nut: unbleached wheat flour, cooked Great Northern white beans and oats, bananas, chia gel, walnuts, yeast, sea salt, unprocessed honey, and bourbon vanilla.

Cocoa Bean: Unbleached wheat flour, cooked Great Northern white beans and oats, chia gel, Dutch-processed cocoa powder, yeast, sea salt, and unprocessed honey.

Pumpkin Lentil: unbleached wheat flour, cooked oats, pumpkin, cooked lentils, chia gel, yeast, sea salt, and unprocessed honey.

Sweet Peach: unbleached wheat flour, cooked Great Northern white beans and cooked oats, chia gel, yeast, sea salt, unprocessed honey.

Lentil Sweet Potato: unbleached white flour, cooked lentils and oats, chia gel, yeast, sea salt, and unprocessed honey.

Chia Maize: unbleached white flour, cooked soy beans and oats, whole corn, chia gel, yeast, sea salt, turmeric, and unprocessed honey.

Breads for a High-Stress World

Knowing that many people in this world of high pressure and fast food don't always have time to eat all the best health-giving foods, Linda and Bill designed their bread to provide all of the eight essential proteins (every one derived from plants and, therefore, low in fat and without cholesterol). Various vegetables and fruits offer nutrients and distinctive natural colors.

Linda and Bill ship their bread and pasta starter base nationwide in the form of frozen ingredients—everything but flour and yeast. It comes with simple instructions on storing, thawing, and baking.

Other Products

One of Linda and Bill's related products, Chia Boost Formula, is also gaining national attention. This is a wholesome, tasty snack product that, unlike its competitors, contains no refined sugar. Each snack is a gel pack, drink, or fruit stick sweetened with natural fruit juices, grade B or C maple syrup, lemon, and cayenne pepper. It is an ideal product for athletes who want quick and lasting energy or people on a weight-loss diet.

Relative to weight control, chia gel is an ideal replacement for fat. Linda says that "one of chia seed's greatest values is as a 'fat replacer.'

"There are 110 recognized fat replacers, and chia seed is not yet on that list. This is a benefit of chia seed that doesn't need clinical studies. All that needs passing is the taste test. We know that when we double the volume of a high-fat salad dressing or spread with chia gel that's ninety percent water, that we have slashed calories by almost one-half.

"We have done blindfold tests with many people, ninety-five percent of whom picked the chia product as the one that tasted better to them. We believe that this is because the saturated chia seed doesn't soak up any juices or flavor, but adds surface area for sensory appeal with a greater texture.

"The same goes for reducing sugars in most jams and jellies, syrups and other flavorings, as well as sauces. This is particularly important for diabetics. Having little flavor of its own—only a mild, nutty taste—chia gel can be used more extensively than prune puree, today's most popular fat replacer."

The next chapter will include tested chia recipes, some of which Linda Barrett and Bill Anderson obtained from venerable Native Americans and others that they designed in their research and development kitchen. They will also be writing a chia recipe book.

Creativity with Chia Seed

Many more chia products will soon emerge from their creative kitchen. Inasmuch as they are proprietary at this time, we cannot mention them. However, there is a vast spectrum of products that imaginative people can devise with chia.

Like what?

How about a chia pancake and waffle mix, chia tortilla, chia salsa, salad dressings, tartar sauce, mustards, dips, jams and jellies, protein drinks, smoothies, milkshakes, malts, yogurt, or a full range of candies, cookies, honeyed sweet rolls, coffee cakes, and cakes? Bill and Linda offer recipe consultation on nutritional enhancement.

Animals thrive on chia seed. One horse trainer reported to chia-grower Bob Andersen that chia meal can combat "sand-belly."

When horses eat grass or other vegetation in beach or desert areas, they ingest much sand that they can't throw off in wastes. Chia seed helps to correct this condition and offers the bonus benefit of making the animals' coats more shiny, due to its high content of essential fatty acids, something veterinarians should know.

Bill and Linda have designed chia recipes for super-nutritious pet foods, especially for dogs. Not only is chia seed going to the dogs, it is also going to the chickens. Ever since the cholesterol scare over eating eggs (unwarranted, as shown by numerous studies, except for the one individual in five hundred who has familial hypercholesterolemia) egg producers have tried to replace some egg saturated fats with unsaturated omega-3 fatty acids. Omega-3 oil has been shown to lessen the risk of heart attack.

By trial and error—equal amounts of both—egg producers have added fish meal, purslane, or flax to the feed for laying hens to increase their intake of omega-3 fatty acids. These supplements succeeded in raising the unsaturated fat content of eggs, but they brought with them an offensive taste or smell that turned off consumers. Further, the eggs had a much shorter shelf life.[4]

So two biochemists, Wayne Coates of the University of Arizona in Tucson and Ricardo Ayerza of the University of Catamarca in Argentina, tried another supplement: chia seed.

Substituting thirty percent chia seed for the usual feed offered at a commercial egg company, they found that the chickens ate with greater gusto and produced the usual number of eggs that looked, tasted, and smelled like conventional eggs and had a comparable shelf life.

Further, these eggs proved to be heart-friendly, with twice the ratio of polyunsaturated fats to unsaturated fats. Mission accomplished. Some egg producers have picked up on this research, adding chia seed to chicken feed and selling eggs high in omega-3 fatty acids.[5]

Chia Seed: Versatile Beyond Versatility

And speaking of eggs, gelatinous, dissolved chia seeds can be used as an egg substitute for cooking and baking. Chia gel can be used to double the volume of salad dressings and cut calories by fifty percent, while adding a greater texture for the best salads. It can also be used to thicken gravies and soups.

It is best not to eat chia seeds dry, because they have a dehydrating effect. Prevent this effect by drinking plenty of fluids with them. Chia seed can be cold-pressed into salad oils and oils for cooking.

It can be added to honey for food value enrichment. Chia is a natural for providing fiber for those troubled with lazy bowel movement. An unlimited number of sports products can be designed to rev up the energy and endurance of athletes.

Inasmuch as chia seed contains far more calcium than milk per gram, some persons, particularly the milk-intolerant, substitute chia for milk and mix the gel into bread dough, hot cereals, and soups. Some use chia seed gelatin in place of egg white.

Gelatinous chia seed is ideal for blending into the dough for baking corn chips and for extending nut butters. With its high content of chlorogenic acid, caffeic acid, and flavonol glycosides, chia gel is an ideal antioxidant to add to prepackaged food products.

It can also be mixed with fruit juice, plain water, or yogurt. Taking a cue from ancient Mayas and Aztecs, a person could devise a vast assortment of beverages from gelatinous chia. In Mexico, people still mix the gelatinous chia seeds into orange or lime or lemon/lime juice—the latter two sweetened with honey. Chilled, this is a refreshing and nourishing drink.

Way Beyond Food Uses

Aside from its use in food, chia oil can be added to cosmetics. Chia's high amount of dietary fiber—especially the soluble form—is important as a source of gum-thickener for use in cosmetics.

Some entrepreneurs are already contemplating deriving and selling chia oil for furniture polishes and antiquing. Following the ancient Aztecs, others are planning to use oil of chia as a preservative coating to keep paintings from oxidizing and losing color from exposure to light over the years.

Inasmuch as chia is a food established by native populations over the centuries, some entrepreneurs are considering it for medicinal products. Certainly, chia could furnish the base for many food pharmacological products. The prospects for food, beverage, cosmetic, and other uses of chia are only as unlimited as one's imagination!

Food distributors and health food stores interested in ordering chia seed can find the source nearest them by con-

tacting Earth Products by phone at (760) 727-9764 or email at
randersn@connectnet.com.

CHAPTER 12

Recipes Using Chia Seed

THE FOLLOWING RECIPES WERE CREATED FOR THIS BOOK BY Linda Barrett and William "Bill" Anderson, cofounders of Menu 4 Life. We are using them with their permission and our thanks. They are producing and testing recipes for an even more comprehensive chia seed recipe book.

Beyond the recipes that follow, chia seed may be used in hundreds of ways as an ingredient in many recipes, from entrees, to snacks, to sauces and desserts, in bakery goods and cooked foods. Shift your creativity into high gear and let it run!

When prepared, chia seed is more than ninety percent water. When saturated with water it has a tapioca-like consistency, which makes it blend well with most other foods.

Because it has such a high water content, it is low in calories. In its saturated or gel form, it can be added to spreads such as mayonnaise, salad dressings, peanut butter, yogurts, and any dip, as well as to milkshakes, puddings, and to almost any dessert to reduce or displace a lot of calories.

Chia seed gel is a great extender. Mayonnaise can be doubled in volume by adding an equal amount of prepared chia gel. Added to a spread such as butter, it reduces calories by forty-five percent per total volume. Further, it brings a delicious texture from its water-soluble fiber or gel.

In gel form, chia can be added to hot cereals such as oatmeal, cornmeal, and whole wheat, and to hot cakes, waffles, and the batter for French toast. It is great in bread puddings.

Dry chia seed will absorb seven times its weight in water. If a dehydrated person eats dry chia seed, it will draw water from his or her body and could form a blockage in the colon. Water saturated chia seeds are also called "prepared" seeds. These will keep for up to three weeks in the refrigerator.

To make "prepared chia gel," always mix dry chia seeds into water while stirring rapidly with a wire whisk. Never pour water into dry seeds, because they will clump. Mix one part chia into ten parts water. For example, add ¼ cup dry chia to 2½ cups water. Let stand 5 minutes and mix again. Allow to set up for at least 15 minutes. Keep refrigerated for use in recipes.

Chia gel is ideal for use in breads of all kinds. Bread dough containing chia gel can be prepared in advance and frozen for future use. Muffins can use 1 to 2 teaspoons each, and cookies, ½ to 1 teaspoon per 2-inch cookie.

Soups

Big Bill's Mushroom Soup

 1 pound mushrooms, 3 varieties, if possible, whole or chopped
 2 tablespoons butter
 1 onion, chopped and sautéed
 2½ cups milk or nut milk (such as cashew or almond)
 (Blend ½ cup raw nuts to 2 cups hot water in blender. Always
    wash raw cashews thoroughly in hot water before using.)
 ½ teaspoon sweet basil
 2 cloves garlic, diced
 2 stalks celery, finely chopped
 1 medium tomato, diced
 1 teaspoon soy or tamari sauce
 ½ teaspoon salt
 ¼ teaspoon cayenne pepper
 ½ cup chia gel

❖❖❖

Saute chopped onions in butter until lightly browned. Mix all
ingredients, except tomato, in large saucepan. Heat to boiling.
Turn to medium-low setting and let simmer 20 to 30 minutes.
Add diced tomato and cook 1½ minutes. Add chia gel just
before serving. Serves 5.

Fruit Soup

6 cups fruit, preferably fresh, but canned is okay
1 cup chia gel
2¾ cups fruit juice
3 tablespoons Minute Tapioca
1 teaspoon vanilla
⅓ cup maple syrup

❖❖❖

Add chia gel to fruit and mix well in a large pot. Prepare tapioca by combining fruit juice and tapioca in saucepan. Let stand 5 minutes. Cook over medium heat until mixture comes to full boil. Remove from heat and let stand 20 minutes. Pour over fruit mixture. Heat to a simmer. Remove from heat. Add vanilla and maple syrup, to taste. Serve over Zwieback. (You can make fresh zwieback overnight by putting your favorite bread slices into an oven set at lowest temperature until dry.) Serves 6.

Christmas Lima Bean Winter Soup

2 cups Christmas lima beans (wash and soak overnight)
8 cups water
½ red bell pepper, chopped
½ green bell pepper, chopped
1 large onion, finely chopped
2 carrots, quartered and finely chopped
2 cloves garlic, finely chopped
2 tablespoons olive oil
½ teaspoon toasted sesame oil
2 tablespoons safflower oil
⅛ teaspoon cayenne pepper
1 tablespoon iodized salt or sea salt
1 teaspoon dried parsley
½ cup chia gel

✢✢✢

Rinse beans and put into a stockpot with 2 quarts of water. Boil 10 minutes. Cook over medium heat until tender, about 30 minutes.

To prepare soup, sauté onions, carrots, garlic, cayenne, and parsley in oil over medium heat for 3 minutes. Add sauté mix, salt, red and green bell peppers, and chia to beans and cook for 20 minutes. Serves 6.

For a succotash winter soup, add 1 cup fresh or frozen whole corn with ¼ teaspoon of cumin to sauté mix.

Creamy Mushroom Soup

1 pound mushrooms, mixed variety, if possible
1½ tablespoons butter
2 tablespoons safflower oil
1½ medium yellow or Maui onions, diced
1 cup raw cashews, washed thoroughly in hot water)
1½ tablespoons dry chia seed
1½ teaspoons dried sweet basil
2 cloves garlic, diced
2 stalks celery with leaves, diced
1 teaspoon sesame oil
1 teaspoon (scant) tamari
½ teaspoon salt
¼ teaspoon cayenne pepper
1 medium tomato

❖❖❖

Add raw cashews to 5½ cups water and blend until smooth, to make 6½ cups of cashew nut milk. Add chia seed and let stand for 15 minutes. Next, sauté half the mushrooms in safflower oil for 4 minutes. Add nut milk and blend. Pour mix into saucepan. Sauté onion, celery, and garlic in 1 tablespoon oil with basil and tamari for 4 minutes. Add sautéed vegetables to liquid mix. Slice or chop remaining mushrooms and add to mix along with cayenne pepper, sesame oil, and salt. Cook for 15 minutes. Chop tomato and add 1½ minutes before serving. Serves 5.

Mulligatawny Soup

1 cup red lentils
½ teaspoon turmeric
5 cups vegetable stock
1 medium potato, diced
5 cloves garlic, minced
1¼-inch cube finely grated ginger
1¼ cups water
1¼ teaspoons salt
⅛ teaspoon cayenne
3 tablespoons canola oil
1 teaspoon coriander
1 tablespoon lemon juice
3 cups chia gel

❖❖❖

Combine all ingredients except garlic, ginger, lemon juice, coriander, and chia gel. Cook until lentils are done. Add remaining ingredients and cook 10 minutes on simmer. Serve hot. Serves 6.

Snowcap Cream Soup

2 cups Snowcap beans (Soak in 8 cups water overnight, drain
    and rinse.)
7 cups water
½ cup of half-and-half
1½ tablespoons dry chia seed
1 or 2 medium onions, chopped
2 cloves garlic, finely chopped
2 stalks celery, finely chopped
2 carrots, quartered and chopped
½ pound mushrooms, chopped
2 tablespoons fresh parsley
1 teaspoon dried basil
½ red bell pepper, finely chopped
2 tablespoons olive oil
½ teaspoon toasted sesame oil
pinch of cayenne pepper, optional
salt, to taste

Cook beans in water until tender, approximately 1½ hours.
Saute onions, garlic, celery, parsley, basil, and cayenne
pepper in olive oil over medium heat for 5 minutes. Add ½
cup of cooked Snowcap beans to sauté mix. Cook together
for two additional minutes. Pour sauté mix in blender and
puree until smooth. Pour blended mix into remaining beans,
adding half-and-half, mushrooms, carrots, red bell peppers,
sesame oil, and salt. Cook over low heat for 20 minutes, add
chia seed, and let stand for 10 minutes. Serve hot. Serves 8.

Spicy Five Bean Soup

½ cup cranberry beans
½ cup European soldier beans
½ cup Snowcap beans
½ cup black beans
½ cup Appaloosa beans (Soak beans for minimum of 24 hours;
  drain and use as follows.)
3 tablespoons safflower oil
1 tablespoon butter
3 carrots, chopped
2 celery stalks with leaves, finely chopped
1 large onion, diced
3 cloves garlic, finely chopped
½ teaspoon toasted sesame oil
¼ cup fresh parsley, chopped
2 tablespoons dried basil
3 dried bay leaves (leave whole)
1 teaspoon cumin powder
1 tablespoon tamari
3 Hungarian peppers, finely chopped
¼ teaspoon cayenne pepper
1½ tablespoons dry chia seed
salt, to taste

✦✦✦

Place beans in pot. Cover with cold water, 3 inches above
beans. Bring to boil and boil for 10 minutes. Reduce heat,
cover, and simmer for 1 hour. Add water as needed to keep
beans covered by 3 inches. In sauté pan, add oil and butter,
celery, onions, garlic, basil, and Hungarian peppers and sauté
for 4 minutes. Add sauté mix to beans, adding bay leaves,
cumin, cayenne, tamari, sesame oil, salt, and carrots. Cover
and simmer on low heat for ½ hour. Stir in chia seed, cover,
and let stand for 10 minutes. Remove bay leaves and serve
hot. Serves 12.

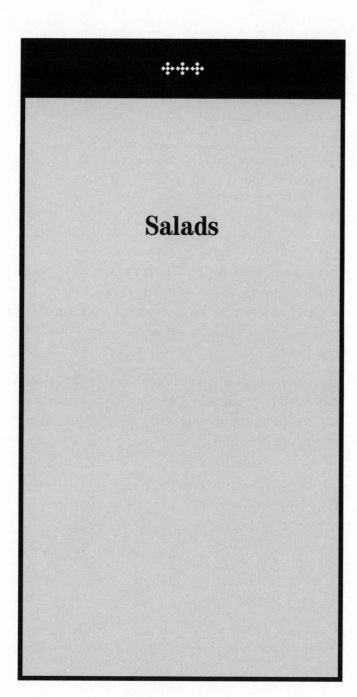

Salads

Coleslaw

1 cup cauliflower tips
1 cup broccoli tips
½ small cabbage, shredded
2 medium carrots, grated
¼ green bell pepper, finely chopped
¼ red, yellow, or orange bell pepper, finely chopped
5 radishes, finely sliced
5 green onions, diced
2 large tomatoes, diced
½ cup chia gel

For extra-crisp coleslaw, place 2-inch chunks of cabbage in blender with a few ice cubes and cover with water. Blend until ¼-inch or smaller pieces of cabbage are formed. Drain in colander and keep refrigerated until ready to mix with other ingredients.

Steam broccoli and cauliflower tips for 5 minutes. Cool in refrigerator 1 hour or drop in ice water for 5 minutes. Mix well into remaining ingredients and top with your favorite salad dressing. Serve chilled. Serves 8.

Rice Salad

   3 cups cooked brown or basmati rice
   2 tablespoons olive oil
   2 tablespoons lemon juice
   1 to 2 cloves garlic, diced
   ½ teaspoon salt
   1 teaspoon fresh diced or (½ teaspoon dried crushed rosemary
      leaves) OR
   1 teaspoon fresh oregano or (½ teaspoon dried oregano)
   ⅛ teaspoon cayenne pepper
   ½ cup chia gel
   1 small zucchini, julienned
   1 medium tomato, seeded and chopped
   2 tablespoons grated Parmesan cheese

❖❖❖

Place rice in a large bowl. Stir in vegetables. Combine oil,
lemon, garlic, salt, herbs, and chia gel in jar and shake well.
Pour over rice mixture. Toss lightly. Cover and chill in
refrigerator for 60 minutes. Serves 6.

Spinach Salad

Dressing:
¼ cup chia gel
⅓ cup low-fat mayonnaise
2 tablespoons honey
1 tablespoon rice or white wine vinegar
½ teaspoon fresh ground black pepper (⅛ teaspoon cayenne
    may be substituted)
¼ teaspoon garlic powder
¼ teaspoon salt
1 tablespoon water

✣✣✣

Whisk dressing ingredients together.

Salad:
¾ pound fresh spinach, washed carefully
2 tomatoes, cut in wedges
2 avocados, cut in cubes
¼ cup mushrooms, thinly sliced
2 hard-boiled eggs, sliced
3 thin slices red onion
¼ cup imitation bacon bits
1 cup croutons

✣✣✣

Arrange above ingredients together on a plate or toss in bowl.
Top with chia dressing and croutons. Serves 5.

Tomato "Sun" Pasta Salad

6 to 8 large tomatoes, diced
1 teaspoon each fresh herbs: basil, oregano, chives, parsley
Pinch of nutmeg
Salt and garlic, to taste
1 roasted, peeled red bell pepper
¼ cup olive oil
½ cup chia gel

❖❖❖

Mix herbs, chia gel, oil, and bell pepper. Puree lightly in blender. Pour over tomatoes and set in the sun in a covered glass bowl 3 to 4 hours. Serve over your favorite chilled pasta. Serves 6.

Main Dishes

Broccoli-Tofu Quiche with Wild Mushrooms

Crust:
2 cups whole wheat pastry flour or barley or brown rice flour
⅓ cup cold-pressed safflower oil
⅓ cup water
¼ teaspoon sea salt

✤✤✤

Mix oil with flour. Add water and mix into a soft dough. Sprinkle flour on surface before rolling out dough to desired thickness and shape.

Filling:
3 to 4 cloves garlic, minced
6 ounces fresh wild mushrooms: shiitake, porcini, chanterelle
6 ounces white button mushrooms
1 tablespoon extra-virgin olive oil
1 teaspoon dry basil
1 teaspoon dry marjoram
1 cup very small broccoli florets
1½ pound soft tofu
2 tablespoons umeboshi vinegar
2 tablespoons cold-pressed sunflower oil
½ teaspoon sea salt, or to taste
½ cup chia gel

✤✤✤

Mix all ingredients and pour into pie shell. Bake 45 minutes in 375-degree oven. Serves 6.

Capellini Alfredo Primavera

½ onion, chopped
¼ green bell pepper, chopped
¼ red bell pepper, chopped
1 large celery stalk, chopped
2 cloves garlic, sliced or minced
2 tablespoons olive oil
½ cup chia gel
1 package Alfredo sauce
1 can cream of mushroom soup
¾ cup fresh, frozen, or canned peas
1 pound capellini pasta, cooked to directions
Basil (fresh or dried), to taste
Oregano (fresh or dried), to taste

❖❖❖

Mix first 7 ingredients and sauté until tender. Add Alfredo Sauce (prepared according to directions), peas, and cream of mushroom soup. Spoon over hot capellini noodles and sprinkle with basil and oregano. Any vegetable may be added or substituted, such as zucchini, carrots, broccoli, cauliflower, corn, or green beans. Serves 6.

Caponata

1 large eggplant, peeled, if desired, and diced
1 large onion, diced
½ pound mushrooms, sliced
1 pound chopped fresh tomatoes (preferably Roma)
3 cloves garlic, minced
¼ cup dry white wine or rice wine vinegar
1 tablespoon olive oil
½ cup chia gel
Oregano (fresh or dried), to taste
Rosemary (fresh or dried), to taste
Salt, to taste

✤✤✤

In a large skillet, heat oil and sauté onion until soft. Add egg-plant and mushrooms. Cook until tender, about 15 minutes. Add water, as needed, to avoid burning. Add tomato, garlic, and wine and continue to cook until very soft. Add chia gel. Season with a little oregano, rosemary, and salt, as desired. Zucchini, red bell peppers, and capers may also be used in this dish. Serves 6.

Corn Cakes

2 tablespoons chia seeds, dry
1 cup yellow or blue corn meal
1 cup potato flour or potato flakes
2 cups vegetable broth
⅓ cup yellow or Maui onion, diced
¼ cup Ortega or Hungarian pepper, diced
2 cloves garlic, minced
⅛ teaspoon cayenne pepper
¼ teaspoon salt, or to taste
¼ teaspoon cumin
½ teaspoon chili powder
Safflower or olive oil to cover skillet bottom

✤✤✤

Place corn meal and potato flour (or flakes) and chia seed in a large bowl. Heat vegetable broth and pour into flour. Mix and set aside. Sauté onion, peppers, garlic, basil, salt, and cumin in lightly oiled skillet over medium heat until tender. Fold sauté mix into corn meal and flour mix. Form dough into approximately 12 patties. Heat enough safflower or olive oil to cover bottom of skillet. Brown chia corn cakes on both sides and serve warm.

Pizza Supreme

Pizza dough, from favorite recipe or ready-made dough
2 tablespoons dry chia seed
2 cups tomato sauce
Toppings (see below)

✛✛✛

Roll out dough into half-inch-thick pizza shape on smooth floured surface. Brush with olive oil (optional). Let rise 20 to 25 minutes. Bake in preheated 375-degree oven for 15 minutes. Take out and cool slightly before topping. (Crust may be frozen for future use, up to 2 months.)

While dough is baking, mix chia seed with tomato sauce. When crust is cool, spread with tomato sauce and your favorite toppings: basil, oregano, sautéed onions, mushrooms, eggplant, broccoli, cauliflower, olives, cabbage, zucchini, hot peppers, artichokes, and whatever else you like. Sprinkle with a little feta cheese, goat cheese, Romano, Parmesan, or mozzarella. (Cheese is optional. Cheeseless vegetarian pizzas are great.) Bake for 15 to 20 minutes in a 425-degree oven. Serve hot.

Vegetable Rice Loaf

1 tablespoon olive oil
½ cup onion, chopped
2 cups carrots, grated
2 cups brown rice, steamed
¼ cup almond or peanut butter
1 cup quick rolled oats
1½ cups vegetable stock or water or 1½ cups soy or regular
   milk
1 teaspoon dry or 4 teaspoons fresh parsley
¼ teaspoon thyme
1 teaspoon sage
1 teaspoon salt
¼ teaspoon onion powder
½ teaspoon garlic powder
¾ cup chia gel

❖❖❖

Sauté onion in oil. Combine all ingredients. Spray nonstick
loaf pan with oil and pour in mixture. Sprinkle with paprika.
Bake at 350 degrees for 45 minutes. Top with garbanzo gravy
(recipe follows).

Garbanzo Gravy

2 cups water
½ onion, chopped and sautéed
4 tablespoons soy sauce or tamari
¼ cup unbleached flour
¾ cup cooked garbanzos, pureed
½ teaspoon salt
⅛ teaspoon celery seed
½ cup chia gel

❖❖❖

Mix all ingredients together, heat to boiling, and serve over Vegetable Rice Loaf or any other vegetable/grain casserole.

George's Mexican Beans

      3 cups pinto beans, cooked
      2 cups soy beans, cooked
      1 large onion, chopped
      1 cup celery, chopped (leaves and all)
      1 large bell pepper, chopped
      4 cloves garlic, minced
      2 tablespoons safflower oil
      2 pounds Ortega salsa (mild, medium, or hot)
      2 teaspoons cumin powder
      1 teaspoon Italian herbs

❖❖❖

Sauté vegetables in oil. (If desired, vegetables may be steamed until tender.) Add cooked beans, cumin powder, herbs, and salsa. Simmer together until vegetables are done, about 20 minutes. Serves 6 to 8.

Sautéed Mushrooms with Polenta

Sautéed Mushrooms:
2 tablespoons unsalted butter
2 tablespoons olive oil
3 shallots, peeled and minced or ⅓ cup minced onion
1 pound any type mushroom, stemmed and thinly sliced
½ cup fresh minced parsley (or 3 tablespoons dry)
⅓ cup chia gel
Salt, to taste

Polenta:
1 quart soup stock (vegetable or meat)
2 cups water
13 ounces coarse cornmeal or polenta
⅔ cup Parmesan cheese

✤✤✤

Heat butter and olive oil together in a large skillet over medium-high heat. Sauté shallots until soft and clear. Add mushrooms and sauté about 5 minutes. Season with parsley and salt. Add chia gel and heat until warm.

To make polenta, bring soup stock and water to a boil in a large saucepan. Slowly sprinkle polenta while stirring with a wire whisk. Cook until thick and soft. Mix chia gel into polenta.

Spoon hot chia polenta onto serving plates and top with a generous portion of sautéed mushrooms. Sprinkle top with Parmesan cheese and serve steaming hot. Serves 8.

Extra polenta may be poured into a dish and refrigerated, to be cut into strips for frying, as you would bacon. Great for breakfast, but good anytime!

Breakfasts

Cinnamon-Orange Pancakes

¾ cup all-purpose flour
1 cup oat flour
2 teaspoons baking powder
1 tablespoon brown sugar
1 teaspoon cinnamon
1 cup skim milk or soy milk
¾ cup orange juice
¾ cup chia gel
1 teaspoon grated orange peel
Vegetable oil spray

In mixing bowl, combine dry ingredients and mix well. In another bowl, combine all liquid ingredients, chia gel, and orange peel. Stir well. Pour liquid ingredients into dry ingredients and stir only until moistened. Preheat griddle. Spray lightly with oil. Ladle batter onto griddle. Turn when bubbles appear. Serve with Orange-Date Syrup (page 130).

Orange-Date Syrup

1 cup boiling water
1 cup pitted dates
¾ cup frozen orange juice concentrate
1 cup chia gel

✤✤✤

Simmer water and dates together and mash. Remove from heat and add orange juice. Whip in a blender. Pour into a quart jar and add chia gel. Shake well. Store in refrigerator. Great over Cinnamon-Orange pancakes.

Pancake Syrup

✤✤✤

Add 1 to 2 teaspoons chia gel to your favorite syrup. Will keep indefinitely in refrigerator.

Peanut Butter-Raspberry Sauce

    4 tablespoons all-natural peanut butter
    ⅔ cup warm water
    4 tablespoons raspberry jam
    ⅔ cup chia gel

✛✛✛

Mix peanut butter and water well in blender. Pour into bowl. Add raspberry jam and chia gel. Mix well with wire whisk. Makes 2 cups sauce.

Raspberry jam may be replaced with 1 banana, 2 apricots (pureed with peanut butter and water), 5 large strawberries, or your favorite fruit.

THE MAGIC OF CHIA

Scrambled Eggs

❖•❖•❖

Mix ½ teaspoon chia gel for each egg, and prepare eggs as usual.

French Toast

❖•❖•❖

Mix 1 to 2 teaspoons chia gel per slice with egg mixture, and prepare as usual.

Vegetable Stir-Fry

½ teaspoon olive oil
1 tablespoon dry chia seed
2 teaspoon ginger root, minced or finely grated
3 large garlic cloves, finely chopped
½ teaspoon toasted sesame oil
3 tablespoons tamari or soy sauce
3 tablespoons rice vinegar
¾ cup water
2 cups kale, coarsely chopped
2 carrots, in thin diagonal slices
⅓ yellow onion, thinly sliced
⅓ red bell pepper, thinly sliced
⅓ green bell pepper, thinly sliced
3 ounces mushrooms, your favorite
2 medium tomatoes, chopped
5 cups cooked brown rice (I prefer brown basmati)

✢✢✢

In a large wok or skillet, sauté garlic and ginger in oils over medium heat until softened (approximately 2 minutes). Add tamari, vinegar, and water and stir-fry for 1 minute. Add vegetables, tomatoes, and chia seeds, cover and cook, stirring occasionally, for 10 minutes or until vegetables are firm yet tender. Serve over rice. Serves 5.

Spicy Atole

Atole is an ancient gruel that was a main part of the Aztec diet. Here's how to make it.

Cornmeal or polenta
Chia gel
Peppers
Honey

❖❖❖

Prepare cornmeal or polenta according to directions on box. Mix 1 to 2 teaspoons chia gel per serving into hot gruel. Add finely chopped jalapeno, chilies or pimiento to gruel.

For a sweet atole, mix 1 to 2 teaspoons honey into gruel instead of peppers. This gruel may be poured into a mold, chilled in the refrigerator overnight, sliced, and cooked like bacon strips in oil or butter.

Breadings, Sauces, Dressings, Salads, and More

Breading

2 cups wheat flour (unbleached or whole wheat)
3 tablespoons dry chia seed
1 tablespoon dry basil
Pinch tarragon
1 teaspoon salt, or to taste
1 teaspoon dill
3 eggs (or 4 egg whites)
6 ounces beer
¼ to ½ teaspoon cayenne pepper (optional)

❖❖❖

Mix dry ingredients together. Mix eggs and beer together and whip 2 minutes in blender. Dip vegetables, fish, or chicken, into egg and beer mixture. Roll or shake in dry mix. Shake off excess and place in fryer, on grill, or in oven. Cook or bake at 375 degrees until golden brown.

Suggestions for breading: zucchini, cut in strips or circles; potatoes or sweet potatoes, cut in thin slices or strips; onion rings; broccoli stalks, peeled and cut in circles or strips; cauliflower or broccoli florets; spinach or kale, cut in strips or half-inch circles; mushrooms, whole or cut in half.

Hash Browns

4 large white potatoes or 8 red potatoes
3 tablespoons dry chia seed
½ yellow onion, finely sliced
¼ green bell pepper, diced
¼ red bell pepper, diced
2 cloves garlic, finely diced
½ teaspoon sweet basil
Pinch of cayenne (optional)
Salt, to taste

✢✢✢

Grate potatoes and place in a large bowl containing ¼ cup water. Sprinkle in dry chia seeds, stir together, and let stand 15 minutes. Add rest of ingredients and mix well. Form into patties and place into slightly oiled skillet and cook until golden brown. For spicy hash browns, add 2 Hungarian peppers and 2 Serrano peppers, finely diced. Serves 5.

Curried Potato Salad

12 red potatoes, boiled and chopped
1 red or yellow onion, chopped
½ green bell pepper, chopped
½ red bell pepper, chopped
2 Hungarian peppers, finely chopped
1 Serrano pepper, finely chopped
½ bunch Italian parsley, finely chopped
1 cup celery, finely chopped
1 package soft tofu
½ teaspoon mustard
1½ teaspoon curry powder
½ teaspoon cumin powder
½ teaspoon cayenne pepper (optional)
¼ teaspoon salt, or to taste
¼ cup olive oil
¼ cup chia gel

❖·❖·❖

Combine potatoes, onion, peppers, parsley, and celery. Whip oil with tofu in a blender. Add spices and chia gel and continue to whip until smooth. Mix all ingredients together and serve.

Greek Red Potatoes au Gratin

1 pound unpeeled red potatoes, sliced
1 large onion, sliced
½ cup feta cheese
⅓ cup unbleached flour
½ teaspoon dry Greek oregano or 1½ teaspoon fresh
½ cup evaporated milk
1 teaspoon olive oil
½ cup chia gel

✠✠✠

In a shallow 2-quart greased baking dish, layer half the potatoes, onions, feta, and oregano. Make a second layer. Mix chia gel with evaporated milk and pour over potatoes. Drizzle with olive oil. Bake 1 hour at 375 degrees or until potatoes are tender. Serves 6.

Fruit Salad

3 peaches, diced
2 apples, diced
2 cups seedless grapes
2 cups pineapple, diced
2 bananas (separate into thirds by running fingers lengthwise
    through center of banana, then dice in small pieces)
2 cups Chia "Sunshine" Sauce (recipe follows)
½ large lemon
2 to 3 tablespoons maple syrup, or to taste

Mix diced fruit occasionally while dicing to prevent browning
of fruit. Juice lemon over fruit for same purpose. Spoon Chia
"Sunshine" Sauce over individual servings. Serves 6.

Chia "Sunshine" Sauce

    1 large mango
    2 bananas
    ½ cup chia gel
    2 tablespoons maple syrup

✤✤✤

Blend fruit in blender until creamy. Mix chia gel into fruit with a spoon.

Apple-Pear Sauce

2 tablespoons chia seed, dry
3 Pippin apples, peeled
5 Gala, Golden Delicious, or Gravenstein apples, peeled
3 Bartlett pears, peeled
¼ cup maple syrup, grade C, if possible
¼ cup turbinado sugar
½ teaspoon cinnamon
Pinch nutmeg (optional)
Juice of 1 to 2 limes, or to taste
½ cup Cranapple juice

✥✥✥

Dice apples and pears. Mix together all ingredients in saucepan. Cook until tender, approximately 25 minutes. Serve warm.

Moroccan Carrot Salad

8 carrots, cut to matchstick size
3 cloves garlic, minced
1 teaspoon cumin
¼ teaspoon white pepper or ⅛ teaspoon cayenne pepper
2 tablespoons olive oil
¼ cup chia gel
Fresh parsley, to taste
Salt, to taste
Crushed red pepper, to taste
Sesame seeds, for garnish

✛✛✛

Sauté carrots over medium heat in a little water until semi-crisp. Drain well. Add olive oil and seasonings, toss, and serve. Makes 4 to 6 servings.

Zippy Salad Dressing

1 cup mayonnaise
½ cup tomato juice
½ cup chia gel
1 teaspoon parsley
1 teaspoon chives
¼ teaspoon garlic salt
¼ teaspoon celery salt

Shake all ingredients in a jar, or mix well with a whisk. Use over your favorite salads.

Children's Recipes

Chips

✤ ✤ ✤

Spray a clean cookie sheet (preferably nonstick) with a light
coat of oil. Spoon chia gel by the teaspoon onto cookie sheet,
three inches apart. Place pan in oven at lowest setting, 170
degrees or lower, and leave overnight or for at least 12 hours.
The dry chips, which resemble potato chips, may be
sprinkled lightly with salt, garlic salt, or any herb seasoning.
This is a high-energy food!

Fruit Pops

✛✛✛

Mix 1 teaspoon chia gel per pop into fruit juice or fresh fruit puree. Spoon into frozen pop mold. Let set in freezer overnight or for at least 4 hours. A great low-fat, high-energy frozen pop for hot summer days.

Dessert Pops

✛✛✛

Blend frozen yogurt or your favorite dairy blend with 1 teaspoon of chia gel per pop. Spoon into pop mold. Let set at least 4 hours in freezer.

Peanut Butter

❖❖❖

Mix equal parts prepared chia seeds with peanut butter (chunky or smooth, preferably natural, not extended with hydrogenated vegetable oil). Mix rapidly with a fork until it turns creamy white.

Makes great peanut butter and jelly sandwiches that won't stick to the roof of your mouth! Note: Prepare this peanut butter spread just before making your sandwiches. It does not keep well.

Cream Cheese

❖❖❖

Replace peanut butter in above recipe with cream cheese.

Dried Fruit Jam

❖❖❖

Any dried fruit may be used: apples, apricots (unsulphured preferred), dates, peaches, pears, pineapple. Add just enough water to cover the dried fruit. Simmer until soft or just soak overnight. Put in blender and whip until smooth. Add ¼ cup prepared chia gel to each cup of fruit puree. Adding dates to fruit will increase sweetness. Jam will keep in refrigerator for about 2 weeks or may be frozen for up to 6 months.

Chia gel may be added to any jam or jelly recipe. Add approximately 3 tablespoons per cup of fruit.

Desserts

Carob Fudge

¾ cup maple syrup
1 cup peanut butter (with nonhydrogenated oil)
1 teaspoon vanilla
1 cup almonds, chopped or ground
1 cup walnuts, chopped
½ cup sesame seeds
¼ cup dry chia seeds
½ cup sunflower seeds
½ cup carob powder

✥✥✥

Mix maple syrup, peanut butter, and vanilla. Add carob powder a little at a time. Mix until well blended. Mix all nuts and seeds together and add slowly to carob mixture. Press firmly onto a lightly oiled pan. Refrigerate at least 1 hour. Cut into squares and serve chilled. Must be stored in refrigerator or may be frozen. Makes 24 pieces. A high-energy treat!

Chocolate Mousse

1 pint whipping cream
½ cup Nutella (hazelnut-chocolate spread)

❖❖❖

Whip cream until it forms soft peaks. Add Nutella and whip until firm. Fold in chia gel. Spoon into dessert glasses. Top with chia whipped cream and garnish with macadamia nuts. Serve chilled. Serves 6.

Alternately, the mixture of cream, Nutella, and chia gel may be spooned into popsicle holders and frozen for a delicious frozen pop.

Jello

✣✣✣

Chia gel may be added to any favorite gelatin mold recipe. Add ½ cup chia gel to each six ounces of dry gelatin mix.

Colored chia gel can make an interesting dessert. Mix 4 ounces concentrated Welch's grape juice, 1 ounce water, and 1 ounce dry chia seed. Mix well with wire whisk. Spoon into mold. Let stand 1 hour, mixing occasionally.

Colored chia seeds may also be used in ice cubes to make a conversation-piece drink.

Cookies

✣✣✣

Add chia gel to any cookie batter for extra energy. Mix in about ½ cup chia gel per dozen cookies, and follow usual baking directions.

Puddings

✣✣✣

Add 1 teaspoon or more of chia gel to each serving of your favorite pudding. Just mix it in with a spoon. Adds great texture! Enjoy!

Crunchy Icebox Pudding

    4 cups corn flakes
    ¼ cup brown sugar or maple syrup
    1 teaspoon grated orange rind
    1 teaspoon vanilla
    1 cup dates, finely cut
    ½ cup raisins
    ⅓ cup milk or nut milk
    1 cup unsweetened coconut
    1 cup chia gel
    Dash of salt

✠✠✠

Crush corn flakes and set aside ½ cup. To remaining crumbs add salt, sugar, rind, dates, raisins, and coconut and mix well. Mix milk, vanilla, and chia gel together and pour into fruit mixture. Place mixture onto wax paper in two sections. Shape into rolls, approximately 6 inches long and roll in remaining corn flake crumbs. Wrap each roll in wax paper and freeze for 2 hours or refrigerate overnight. Slice in ½-inch pieces. Makes 24 pieces.

Space Balls

3 cups almonds, ground
¾ cup lecithin
½ cup cashew butter
1 cup unsweetened coconut
½ cup currants
2 teaspoons Tahitian or other vanilla
4 tablespoons dry chia seed
½ cup honey
½ teaspoon salt
1½ cups unsweetened coconut for coating

Mix all ingredients together in a large bowl. Knead with your hands until well blended. Press a small handful together firmly, then roll into a ball and roll in dry coconut to coat. These are an excellent gift when placed in a decorative tin. Makes 20 to 30 pieces.

Yummy Granola

2½ cups whole wheat flour
2 cups quick oats
½ cup sunflower seeds
½ cup cashews, raw (wash cashews well under hot water)
½ cup sesame seeds
1 cup corn meal
1 cup rye flour
1 cup wheat germ
1 cup coconut
¾ cup canola oil (or ¼ cup for less fat)
1 cup nonfat powdered milk or soy milk powder
1 cup water
¾ cup maple sugar
1⅓ cup chia gel

✜✜✜

Combine all dry ingredients and mix well. Add water, chia, oil, and maple sugar. Mix and crumble with fingers. Put into shallow pan and bake at 225 degrees for 1½ hours (a little longer for a toasty flavor). Makes 10 cups.

Whipped Cream

❖❖❖

Add 1 to 2 teaspoons chia gel to 1 cup whipped cream. Fold in with a spoon.

Pie Filling

❖❖❖

Chia gel may be added to your favorite fruit or cream pie. Add 1 to 2 teaspoons per serving to pie filling. This will help to reduce calories and add extra nutrients and fiber.

References

Preface

1. Harrison Doyle, personal communication with Bob Andersen.
2. Jan Barstad, *Oil of Chia* (Apache Junction, Ariz.: Jojoba Growers & Processors, Inc., 1990), p. 2.
3. Frey Barnardino de Sahagun, *Florentine Codex*, Book 2, 1558, p. 181.

CHAPTER 1: The Secret Is Out

1. Jane E. Brody, "To Preserve Their Health and Heritage, Arizona Indians Reclaim Ancient Foods," *New York Times*, May 21, 1991.

CHAPTER 2: Chia: A Seed of Greatness

1. Harrison Doyle, personal communication with Bob Andersen.
2. Clyde Hogan, interview with James F. Scheer, April 1996.

CHAPTER 3: Natural Food: The Early Years

1. Keith A. Tucker, "Chia—The Space Age Food," *Let's Live*, May 1964, p. 57.
2. Paul Bragg, lecture, September 1964.

CHAPTER 4: Chia Folk Medicine

1. Harrison Doyle, personal communication with Bob Andersen.
2. Morton Walker, "Pregnancy Requires Omega-3 EFAs," *Health Foods Business*, September 1995, pp. 30, 85.

3. Ibid.

4. Jay Lombard, M.D., and Carl Germano, *The Brain Wellness Plan* (New York: Kensington Books, 1997), p. 44.

5. Ibid., p. 73.

6. Michael T. Murray, N.D., "Research Report: Flaxseed: Nature's Best Source of Omega-3 Oils and Lignans," *Health Counselor,* vol. 6, no. 5, 1995.

7. Mary Clarke, Ph.D., "Eating Fat, Then and Now," Special Report, Kansas State University, 1996.

8. William Lands, Ph.D., "Omega-3 Fatty Acid Studies Hindered by U.S. Diet Rich in Omega-6," *F-D-C Reports—The Tan Sheet,* April 25, 1994.

9. Robert Kleiman, interview, May 1996.

10. Ralph Holman, "Essential Fatty Acids and Nutritional Disorders," *Lipids in Modern Nutrition,* ed. M. Horisburger and U. Bracco, (New York: Vevey/Raven Press), pp. 157–162.

CHAPTER 5: More Chia Folk Medicine

1. Harrison Doyle, personal communication with Bob Andersen.

2. James Hart and William L. Cooper, "Vitamin E in the Treatment of Prostate Hypertrophy," *Lee Foundation for Nutritional Research,* Report #1, November 1941, pp. 1–10.

3. Roger Windsor, "Solving the Mystery of Multiple Sclerosis," *Spectrum,* May/June 1993, p. 11.

4. Ibid.

5. Ibid.

6. Jean Carper, *The Food Pharmacy* (New York: Bantam Books, 1988), pp. 57–58.

7. Gene A. Spiller, "The Facts on Fiber," *Veggie Life,* May 1996, p. 12.

8. Ibid.

9. Tucker, "Chia: The Space Age Food," p. 57.

CHAPTER 6: The Inside Story

1. H.S. Gentry, et al, "Experimental Propagation & Evaluation of Chias for Desert Crops," National Science Foundation, 1993, p. 2.

2. Ibid., p. 4.

3. Ibid.

4. Ibid.

5. G.O. Burr and M.M. Burr, "On the Nature of the Fatty Acids Essential in Nature," *Journal of Biology and Chemistry,* 1930, 86: 587–621.

6. David F. Horrobin, "Gamma Linoleic Acid in Medicine," *1984–85 Yearbook of Nutritional Medicine,* (New Canaan, Ct.: Keats Publishing, Inc., 1985), p. 23–25.

7. Ibid.

8. Ibid.

9. Stephen Langer, M.D. and James F. Scheer, *Solved: The Riddle of Illness* (New Canaan, Ct.: Keats Publishing, 1995), p. 71.

10. Robert Kleiman, personal communication.

11. James Brown, "Chia Markets," 1996 report of International Flora Technologies, Ltd., Apache Junction, Arizona.

12. Ibid.

13. Ibid.

14. Ibid.

15. J.I. Rodale, *The Complete Book of Minerals for Health* (Emmaus, Pa.: Rodale Books, Inc., 1972), pp. 612–613.

16. Michael Colgan, Ph.D., *Optimum Sports Nutrition: Your Competitive Edge* (Ronkokona, N.Y.: Advanced Research Press, 1993), pp. 205ff.

17. Frank Murray, *The Big Family Guide to All Minerals* (New Canaan, Ct.: Keats Publishing, Inc., 1995), p. 237.

18. Ibid.

19. "Boron Found to Have Role in Hardening Bones," *Chemical Marketing Reporter,* November 9, 1987.

20. Judy McBride, "Boron: A New Essential Element," *Scientific Research News,* USDA, April 1989.

21. Ibid.

22. Murray, *The Big Family Guide to All Minerals,* p. 23.

23. Robert M. Giller and Kathy Matthews, *Natural Prescriptions* (New York: Carol Southern Books, 1997), pp. 20, 22, 245, 247.

24. Richard L. Travers, "Boron and Arthritis: The Results of a Double-Blind Pilot Study," *Journal of Nutritional Medicine,* 1990; vol. 1: 127–132.

25. Judy McBride, "Diets Deficient in Boron Can Dull the Senses," USDA News Feature, April 19, 1990.

CHAPTER 7: Seed Foods: The Buffer Against Cancer

1. Walter Troll, Ph.D., personal communication, 1996.

2. Carper, *The Food Pharmacy,* p. 66.

3. Ann Kennedy, "Anticarcinogenic Activity of Protease Inhibitors," in *Protease Inhibitors as Cancer Chemotherapeutic Agents,* ed. Troll and Kennedy (New York: Plenum Press, 1993), pp. 6–7.

4. Ibid, p. 15.

5. Carper, *The Food Pharmacy,* pp. 68–69.

6. Pelayo Correa, "The Epidemiological Approach to the Study of Protease," in *Protease Inhibitors as Cancer Chemopreventive Agents,* p. 6.

7. Ibid., p. 7.

8. Kennedy, *Protease Inhibitors as Cancer Chemopreventive Agents,* p. 55.

9. Ibid.

10. Walter Troll, personal communication, April 1996.

11. "Record-Breaking Ancient Seed Sprouts," Associated Press, August 7, 1972.

12. Bob Andersen, personal communication, April 1997.

13. H. Davidson, et al, "Chemical Composition of Rice in Relation to Soil Fertility in China and Japan," *Science,* 1932, vol. 75, p. 294.

14. R.C. Collison, "Proportion of Organic to Inorganic Minerals in Seeds and Plant Stems and Leaves," *Journal of Industrial and Engineering Chemistry,* August 1912, in J.I. Rodale, *The Complete Book of Food and Nutrition* (Emmaus, Pa.: Rodale Books, 1961), p. 319.

15. Thomas H. Mather, *Scientific Agriculture,* vol. 10, 1929 in *The Complete Book of Food and Nutrition,* p. 320.

16. Ibid.

CHAPTER 8: Domesticating the Wild Chia

1. Bob Andersen, interview

CHAPTER 9: Real Foods for Real People

1. Gary Nabhan, "Native Foods of Desert Peoples Found to Control Diabetes," *The Seedhead News,* Fall 1987.
2. Ibid.
3. "An Ancestral Cure for a Modern Disease," *Vegetarian Times,* October 1990.
4. Jane E. Brody, "To Preserve Health and Heritage."
5. Nabhan, "Native Foods of Desert People."
6. John Willoughby, "Primal Prescription," *Eating Well,* May/June 1991.
7. Weston A. Price, D.D.S., *Nutrition and Physical Degeneration,* sixth ed. (New Canaan, Ct.: Keats Publishing, 1998).

CHAPTER 10: Back to the Past

1. Jane E. Brody, "To Preserve Their Health and Heritage."
2. Ibid.
3. Kevin Dahl, "Ancient Seeds for Modern Needs: The Native Seeds/SEARCH Story," *Seedhead News,* Spring 1991.
4. Willoughby, "Primal Prescription."
5. Somasundaram Addanki, "Roles of Nutrition, Obesity and Estrogen in Diabetes Mellitus," *Preventive Medicine,* 1981: vol. 10: 577–589.
6. Dahl, "Ancient Seeds for Modern Needs."
7. Ibid.
8. Gary Nabhan, "Native Foods and Diabetes Project Takes Off," *Seedhead News,* Fall 1990.
9. "Cactus Foods Help Diabetics," pamphlet of Native Seeds/SEARCH (n.d.).

CHAPTER 11: Creativity with Chia

1. Linda Barrett and William Anderson, frequent interviews.
2. Stephen Schoenthaler, Ph.D., Walter Doraz, and James Wakefield, Jr., "Impact of Low Food Additives and Sucrose Diets on Academic Performance in 803 New York City Public Schools,"

International Journal of Biosocial Research, vol. 8, no. 2, 1986, pp. 185–195.

3. Irwin Rosenberg, M.D., et al, "Link Between Nutrition and Cognitive Development for Children," Report for Nutritional Cognitive National Advisory Committee, 1998.

4. Janet Raloff, "Chia for Your Pet—If It Clucks," *Science News,* April 4, 1998.

5. Ibid.

CHAPTER 12: Recipes Using Chia Seed

1. Recipes by Linda Barrett and William Anderson are used with their permission.

Recipe Index

Index

About the Author

JAMES F. SCHEER IS PAST EDITOR OF THREE HEALTH AND nutrition magazines—*Let's Live, Food-Wise,* and *Health Freedom News.* The author of twenty-two published books, many in the field of nutrition, he wrote the best-sellers *Solved: The Riddle of Illness* with Stephen Langer, M.D., and the million-seller *Foods That Heal* with Maureen Salaman.

More than two thousand of his articles and columns have appeared in a hundred national magazines. One of his non-health books served as the basis for *The Race for Space,* a sixty-minute documentary that was nominated for an Academy Award and was voted winner in its category at the San Francisco International Film Festival.